Also by Mark Elliott Miller...

Extraordinary Encounters in An Ordinary Life (2002)

Advice for Life From the Mouths of Elders:
One Hundred Ways to Grow Old Gracefully (2003)

The Husband's Guide to Cancer Survival (2004)

The Hundred Grand Lesson, A spiritual guide
for men who have lost a relationship and are
contemplating on-line dating (2007).

Doc Miller's Prison Prognosis

An Insider's Examination of Correctional Healthcare

Mark Elliott Miller, MPH

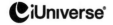

DOC MILLER'S PRISON PROGNOSIS: AN INSIDER'S EXAMINATION OF CORRECTIONAL HEALTHCARE

iUniverse books may be ordered through booksellers or by contacting:

iUniverse
1663 Liberty Drive
Bloomington, IN 47403
www.iuniverse.com
844-349-9409

ISBN: 978-1-6632-4986-9 (sc)
ISBN: 978-1-6632-4987-6 (e)

Library of Congress Control Number: 2023900767

Print information available on the last page.

iUniverse rev. date: 01/17/2023

Contents

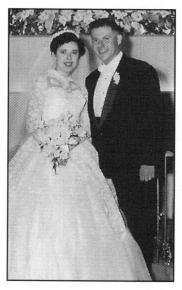

Louise and Hugh Miller, 1955

Dedicated to the memory of my father, Hugh Marvin Miller (1932 - 2004) and mother, Louise Dorothy Miller (1934 - 1989). As a Texas trial attorney, he was a beacon of hope for people from all walks of life. As a father, he modeled how to treat others with respect and to always speak truthfully. As a mother of five, social worker and paralegal, she taught me to love and respect friends and neighbors alike, and share our gifts with the less fortunate.

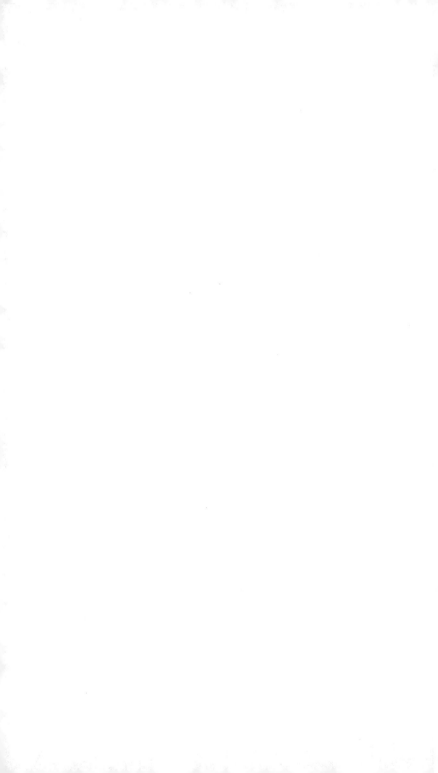

"When the prison gates slam behind an inmate, he does not lose his human quality; his mind does not become closed to ideas; his intellect does not cease to feed on a free and open interchange of opinions; his yearning for self-respect does not end; nor is his quest for self-realization concluded. If anything, the needs for identity and self-respect are more compelling in the dehumanizing prison environment."

— *U.S. Supreme Court Justice Thurgood Marshall*

Chapter 1

Time Served Among
Felons & Friends

Introduction

Welcome to my life in prison. Not as a convicted felon, but as a health services administrator (HSA) overseeing the medical care of thousands of men and women arrested and convicted of drug crimes, driving under the influence, sexual abuse, theft, murder and other violations of law. This was an unusual professional choice for me that followed more traditional work in hospitals, hospices, and rehabilitation centers. However, since I believe strongly that all people deserve quality healthcare, this was an opportunity to serve many people who may have received little or no care in the "free world." In addition to lacking adequate health care, many of the inmates with whom I worked lacked even the basic understanding of maintaining their own health and could benefit from health education. As an educator for 10 years, I taught on campuses for universities in Texas and North Carolina and online for Indiana Wesleyan University and South

Georgia State College. While most of us learn from formal education and informal life experiences, others fail to learn the necessary moral lessons, make poor life choices, and wind up in jails and prisons.

My Mentor

One of my earliest mentors in correctional healthcare was Craig Peters, a long-time healthcare administrator in Texas prisons. As a boy, Craig hung out on the streets for much of his childhood in New York with others of his age. His "gang of friends" were a crowd that appeared to be enroute to either an early grave or a lengthy prison sentence. Craig knew that the only way to escape a life of incarceration or premature death was to get away from the negative influences of his friends and get an education. In his early-adult years, while working as a corrections officer, he earned a bachelor's degree in psychology, a bachelor's degree in business administration, and masters' degrees in education and business administration. With the advanced education, he applied for a healthcare leadership position with the University of Texas Medical Branch (UTMB) in Galveston, TX, where he steadily grew professionally. He also married a dentist and they had a family. "It's all about the choices we make," Craig often said. He was living proof of the truth of that statement.

Contrary to Craig's background, I had a typical suburban, middle class Caucasian upbringing as one of five children to an attorney father and social worker mother. My parents were children of immigrant parents who emphasized education as the impetus for success.

Education served my parents, siblings and me very well. My older brother is a physician, of my younger two brothers one is a teacher and one a commercial real estate appraisal entrepreneur, and my only sister is an attorney. I realize not everyone is as blessed as my family and I do not take that for granted. I have learned from Craig and others on my professional journey that we do have choices, and the choices we make have different results. The defining differences between my life and the lives of men and women in prison is I have a moral foundation built by my nuclear family, the knowledge that I have career options, and the self-discipline to stop, look and listen before making decisions that could affect my trajectory in life. Have these differences allowed me never to act impulsively and make poor choices? Absolutely not. Yet, like Craig, I learned from my mistakes and have grown professionally and spiritually. As a man of integrity, I believe all of us deserve to be mentored as I have been by Craig and others.

Some Background on Prisons

In the chapters ahead, I will take you behind the prison walls and fences in the states where I served as a correctional healthcare administrator. Inside these well-secured places are villages where the residents play board, video, and card games, watch movies and sports on TV, read the Bible, Koran, self-help books and novels, dress in a uniform manner, eat when they are told to eat, sleep when the lights go out, shop when released to the Commissary, and get treated for medical, dental and mental health issues when they need it. Healthcare is one of the few areas of prison life where inmates have some freedom of choice. As wards of the State (and thanks to court challenges to inhumane care in the past) inmates have access to both basic and complex medical, dental and mental health care, regardless of their ability to pay. For most uninsured or underinsured Americans, prison healthcare is often superior to what many of them are able to receive, especially in rural communities and inner-cities that lack an adequate supply of doctors and well-equipped hospitals. However, in some prisons where medical staff recruitment is challenging or driven by private contractors seeking to maximize profits, the care can be poorly delivered or even life-threatening. Over seven years in this field in Texas, Virginia, Georgia and other states, I have had interactions with inmates and co-workers that boggled the mind and inspired me to chronicle some of these experiences here.

Prior to 1976 in America, prison healthcare was often provided by unlicensed staff or inmates assigned to in-house clinics. Doctors and nurses were rarely on-site every day, so correctional officers had no choice but to make emergency healthcare decisions without professional medical guidance. As a result, many lives were lost unnecessarily, triggering lawsuits demanding better prisoner health care. In the landmark Texas lawsuit, Estelle v Gamble (1976), the U.S. Supreme Court ruled in favor of the plaintiff, J.W. Gamble, citing the Eighth Amendment of the Constitution's protection against cruel and unusual punishment. Further case law, Farmer v Brennan (1994), protected inmates from "deliberate indifference to serious medical needs" by healthcare workers in correctional facilities (ultrariskadvisors.com, 10/2011).

Why This Book?

Leading up to my decision to write this book, I left my prison healthcare career in Virginia in December 2020 over patient care differences and decided to take a sabbatical after 34 years in healthcare. At times of crisis, it is good to reconnect with treasured family and friends; so, I donned my cloth mask, boarded a plane, and set out on a two-week trip to visit my family in Texas.

At this time, the COVID Pandemic was spiking once again in diagnosed cases, hospitalizations and deaths. The airlines' mandates clearly communicated, "no mask, no flight" and the airports also required mask wearing in the terminals, but there was very little social distancing evident among the travelers. Most of my flights were fully booked and elbow-to-elbow seating was standard fare, making flying even more uncomfortable and anxiety-causing on these trips than flying coach was in healthier times.

Understandably, the airline industry lost many millions of dollars during the Pandemic when foreign travel was curtailed or eliminated entirely. Foreign flight bans as early as Spring 2020 were good public health policy as one means to reduce COVID case transmission by potentially containing the virus within U.S. borders. Unfortunately, Americans are highly mobile, resulting in even the most isolated parts of our country being affected by COVID. Even though I had studied public health in graduate school at the University of North Carolina-Chapel Hill and understood the realities of this airborne virus, it truly hit home personally and professionally.

I began this book on a plane symbolically to start my story at 30,000 feet. Business leaders often talk about

5

getting a high-level perspective to see the big picture of challenges in their industry before landing at ground level to address it. Also, the healthcare industry where I have worked since 1986 has evolved over the years by learning from the airlines, hospitality industry, Disney and Starbuck's, among others.

I often recall one healthcare industry mantra: "The only constant in healthcare is change." In this book, my fifth in 20 years, I will introduce readers to the healthcare industry in U.S. prisons and jails where I served tens of thousands of incarcerated men and women as a healthcare administrator from 2002 to 2004, 2017 to 2020, and 2021 to this writing in 2023, respectively. Constant change is definitely the norm in correctional healthcare. I hope my experiences will allow you to gain a perspective of correctional healthcare that elicits a greater understanding of a non-traditional area of medical treatment and the fiscal and personal costs associated with it.

Chapter 2

What's Up Doc?

Introduction

Throughout my three decades in healthcare, I have been mistaken numerous times as a doctor because of my well-spoken manner, love of medical science, and rapport with the ill. In the prisons and jails where I have served as a healthcare administrator, correctional officers, staff, inmates, families and attorneys often called me "Doc." From 2002 to 2004, I was employed by the University of Texas Medical Branch-Galveston Correctional Managed Care as healthcare administrator of three prisons in the Houston area, five Dallas County Jail sites, and one State prison in Dallas. From 2017 to 2020, I was employed in the Virginia prison system as a HSA and known as Doc to convicted felons at two male prisons and one women's institution. In 2021 and 2022, I was HSA at a prison in South Georgia and then promoted to be a traveling administrator serving prisons in multiple states. The Doc moniker followed me around the country.

While I have been employed in healthcare administration and higher education for many years, I am not a clinician, but have worked alongside some of the best and the worst doctors, nurses, nurse practitioners and physician assistants in corrections, as well as in hospitals, hospices, home health, rehabilitation centers, and other healthcare entities. I have led and advised healthcare teams in Georgia, Missouri, Montana, Nevada, New Mexico, North Carolina, Oklahoma, South Carolina, Tennessee, Texas, and Virginia. I have never claimed to be a healthcare provider, but have been assumed to be a doctor because I have been mentored through my career by strong clinicians in various disciplines and have a gift for explaining complex medical conditions in terms that patients and their families understand. I also have learned to listen to patients' concerns and show empathy.

The Business of Prison Health Care in Virginia and Texas

The Virginia Department of Corrections (VADOC) leadership spends millions of taxpayer dollars through contractors to operate the majority of its healthcare system. As you can surmise, prison health care in Virginia is big business. The VADOC annual budget for 2021 was $1.39 billion to operate 38 prisons. In Texas, the Department of Criminal Justice (TDCJ) 2021 budget was $3.52 billion to operate 55 prisons, dozens of state jails and other correctional facilities. Comparatively, there were 24,235 inmates in Virginia and over 122,000 people incarcerated in Texas (12/2020 figures). In Virginia, $230 million was spent on inmate care in 2019.

In 2018, Virginia healthcare costs were estimated at $6500 annually per inmate and were the second largest part of the VADOC budget after inmate security and management (Richmond Times-Dispatch, 11/18/18). Fourteen percent of Virginia inmates are at least 55 years old (Richmond Times-Dispatch, 12/19). Most of these older inmates have chronic illnesses that often require costly medications and hospitalizations. In 2019, Texas taxpayers spent over $750 million for prison healthcare, with inmates age 55 and older accounting for 50% of the system's hospitalization costs despite being only 12½% of the prison population. The prison population is increasingly aging (Texas Tribune, 11/25/19).

I worked for two of the three major DOC contractors in Virginia: MedikoPC, a physician-owned company based in Richmond, VA, Armor Health, a privately-held company based in Miami, FL, and the VADOC directly. I did not work for the third contractor, the GEO Group, but found their history interesting.

MedikoPC, a wholly-owned professional corporation led by Iranian-born founder Kaveh Ofogh, MD, has primarily operated jail healthcare and provided psychiatric telemedicine since its founding in 1996. Dr. Ofogh began his company as a staffing agency for physicians interested in correctional healthcare careers and grew it into an operations entity. They were granted contracts for two prisons' healthcare operations in Virginia (Augusta Correctional Center and Coffeewood Correctional Center) when their bid was accepted over Armor Health. However, after five years, Armor regained these prison contracts for a short period of time. Despite losing the prison contracts in Virginia, MedikoPC continued to grow in the Carolinas by serving jails. While the company's owner had an admirable vision driven by a strong immigrant work ethic, they lacked the infrastructure to provide support needed by administrators and clients at prison sites. Turnover was extremely high at the corporate level. I reported to seven regional managers and worked with three corporate medical directors in less than three years. When I was offered a regional manager role by the chief operating officer, I turned it down after Dr. Ofogh refused to explain why there was so little tenure in the position. The answer seemed obvious: If you disagreed with Dr. Ofogh, you were no longer needed. I witnessed this with the departure of Human Resources staff, financial leadership, and Dr. Ofogh's administrative assistant. To his credit, Dr. Ofogh and his company never lost a lawsuit in 24 years of operation.

Armor in Virginia, at this time, was housed within the VADOC headquarters building in Richmond. This was highly unusual since Armor's competitors rented office space in the Richmond metroplex and other areas. They were a few steps or an elevator ride away from the VADOC Health Services Unit (HSU) decision makers every workday. It is well-documented that Armor is no stranger to litigation in Virginia and other states, so this should have failed the smell test of impropriety.

Armor was criminally charged for allegedly falsifying records in the death of a man in Wisconsin and had contracts cancelled by at least seven counties in Colorado, Florida, New York, and Oklahoma. After allegations of failing to meet contractual obligations and placing inmates at risk in New York, the company agreed to pay $350,000 and not bid on any contracts in the state for three years in a 2016 settlement with the New York

Attorney General. Settlements against the company and the counties where it operates have reached into the millions. The family of a 32-year-old New York inmate named Bartholomew Ryan, a former Marine who hanged himself, was awarded $7.8 million. In the Wisconsin case, the family of 38-year-old Terrill Thomas, a Milwaukee father of six who died of dehydration after the water was switched off in his cell and medical staff ignored him, was awarded $6.75 million. The death of Thomas, whose mental illness prevented him from communicating about his lack of water, made national headlines and outraged local leaders. A *New Times* review of court records, news reports, and government documents found at least 34 lawsuits accusing Armor of contributing to a death. In other cases, the inmate survived, but with serious or debilitating injuries. Among them are troubling allegations: In Milwaukee County, a woman gave birth while Armor staff ignored her; the baby died in the same cell where she was born hours earlier. In Oklahoma County, an Armor nurse allegedly tried to perform an exorcism on a woman who was in the throes of drug withdrawal; she died the next day. And in Hillsborough County, Armor staff chose not to send a woman to the hospital after discovering irregularities in an electrocardiogram even though she'd gone into cardiac arrest weeks earlier. The woman, who had been arrested for failing to appear in court while she was in the hospital recovering, died hours after her release from jail. Armor has had contracts in at least 11 states outside their Florida headquarters: Colorado, Georgia, Illinois, Maine, Nevada, New York, Oklahoma, South Dakota, Utah, Virginia, and Wisconsin. Financial statements included in a 2018 Armor bid indicated the company had contract revenues exceeding $242 million in 2017 (Miami New Times, 9/17/19).

The GEO Group, a publicly-traded real estate investment trust based in Boca Raton, FL, has privatized 129 correctional facilities with over 90,000 beds, including one prison in Virginia. The GEO Group spent more than $1.5 million for lobbying in 2019 and contributed over $1.4 million in the 2020 election cycle, including $11,010 to former NC House of Representatives Speaker and current U.S. Senator Thom Tillis (R-NC), $10,000 of which came from the company political action committee, according to campaign finance research group The Center for Responsive Politics. Internationally, GEO operates correctional facilities in Australia, British Columbia, New South Wales, Scotland and South Africa.

Corizon Health, one of the largest investor-owned prison healthcare contractors, no longer provides medical care in Virginia, but in late-2020 still served 149 facilities in 16 states, a decrease in contracts from 534 facilities in 27 states in 2018 (https://www.prisonlegalnews.org, 11/1/20). According to the American Civil Liberties Union, Corizon was sued for malpractice 660 times within five years. Corizon was also fined millions of dollars for inadequate staffing (https://www.prisonlegalnews.org, 3/3/20). On June 30, 2020, the Flacks Group, a Miami-based global investment firm purchased Corizon.

In many cases, these private and publicly-traded companies "treat fines, penalties, settlements and jury awards as merely a cost of doing business—not as a catalyst for change to providing adequate health care" (https://www.prisonlegalnews.org, 3/3/20).

While District Court and U.S. Supreme Court decisions have mandated necessary healthcare reforms that, in theory, lead to more humane treatment, there has also been a shift in corrections philosophies as well. While working in Virginia, I had great admiration for Harold Clarke, the Jamaican-born, VADOC visionary director since 2010, who shifted the prison system from a purely punitive model to a "healing environment" that encouraged education and skill development. He instituted these reforms to reduce recidivism and to enable inmates to earn their Graduate Equivalent Degree (GED) or an associate degree if their incarceration time allowed. I was privileged to attend one graduation ceremony at Coffeewood Correctional Center in Mitchells, VA where diplomas and vocational certificates were awarded to dozens of inmates. The pride these men and their instructors exhibited was palpable.

Educational opportunities for the inmates aside, the VADOC organization is still a paramilitary one where wardens and operational staff micromanage healthcare services in the name of "security" to the detriment of inmates' health. The VADOC HSU has good intentions and clinical expertise, but leaders answer to directors with law enforcement backgrounds and Commonwealth and in-house attorneys instead of the staff closest to the patients. Response to ongoing litigation and fear of further malpractice and civil rights lawsuits are standard operating procedure for the overly cautious VADOC leadership team. Outspoken staff are not welcome in the VADOC HSU world if they find new patient care issues or question authority. I found that bringing quality of care, employee malfeasance and incompetence issues to light, for me was career-limiting.

My Experiences as "Doc"

I love the medical profession, but am increasingly saddened by the growing lack of empathy by many healthcare providers. Correctional nursing, in particular, in the age of COVID, became a money game with "war pay" salary increases through the Pandemic and at least a year following. Nurses traveled across the U.S. wherever they had license reciprocity to work for agencies offering salaries never before seen in the industry. News reports documented traveling nurses working in COVID hot spots like New York and California giving well-deserved rest to hospital staff. Without a doubt, nurses are on the frontlines every day—and in the COVID era, they were under fire! Granted, pandemics are an extremely stressful time to be a nurse and the media's depiction of them as heroes is justified for many, but others lost focus on the patient—what should have motivated them to enter and stay in the profession. All who choose to care for the sick—from paramedic to phlebotomist to nurse to doctor to administrator—deserve to be well-paid, but greed never belongs in healthcare.

I left Virginia in early-2021 to become a HSA for publicly-traded prison owner and operator CoreCivic in South Georgia, and later became a Surge HSA traveling to other states. I witnessed agency nurses and mental health professionals earning wages 40% to 100% higher than staff salaries. Contracts with government entities and care practices mandated specific staffing patterns. Many health professionals dropped out of the workforce following the Pandemic; and in some prisons the agency workers outnumbered staff since there simply were no applicants for open positions. On a positive note, for dedicated healthcare staff, wages increased significantly over this period and leveled the playing field. I believed rates paid by correctional healthcare employers to agencies would slowly decline over time, and saw this occur nationally in the latter half of 2022 as increased wages for staff nursing positions incentivized agency nurses to apply for open jobs. As vacancies decreased, agency pay rates also declined. Since these agencies siphon off as much as 25% of traveling workers' salaries for administrative overhead, they are seeing an end to their market control as many agency workers find a workplace home they can call their own.

There is a well-known cliché in healthcare circles that "nurses eat their young." For readers outside of healthcare, this means experienced nurses often allow new nurses to fail by expecting them to apply in the field what they learned in nursing school without a guiding hand. When the new nurse fails—potentially injuring a patient—they are castigated. Many young nurses drop out of the profession because of the dog-eat-dog nature of the workplace until she or he has proven their competence. It is just too much to bear for often idealistic new nurses; this leads to substandard care based simply on lack of applicable experience. I witnessed a possible cause of this spitefulness. Early in my career, in the 1980's, it was not unusual for some, primarily male, doctors to disrespect and be condescending to nurses working with them in hospitals, surgical suites and other settings. Sexual harassment, from fondling breasts to pats on the butt to coerced sexual encounters occurred, as did doctors throwing scalpels and surgical supplies at nurses and surgical technicians when frustrated. Bitterness from this treatment in the past may have inspired the negativity practiced by some experienced nurses toward their younger peers today. On the other side of the coin, I have seen many nurturing nurses of all ages share their knowledge and generously mentor younger nurses. During my years as a hospice executive director, this was an innate trait exhibited by nurses on my teams.

Another trend I have witnessed is ageism in nursing practice and it flows two ways: Millennial (born between 1981 and 1996) and Gen Z (born between 1997 and early 2000's) staff view Baby Boomers (born between 1946 and 1964) with disdain and create cliques for their own generation, while at the same time older nurses view their younger peers as lacking the maturity, empathy and personal commitment they themselves had 20 to 40 years ago. There are many who work and play well with others (as our kindergarten teachers admonished), but my experience shows that has been the exception rather than the rule in prisons across the United States where infighting, profanity and feelings of entitlement are common.

Medicine in the Time of COVID

During the COVID-19 Pandemic, patients—with or without a COVID diagnosis—deserved consistent, on-going care from their professional caregivers. In too many cases in prisons nationwide, however, treatment of many medical and dental conditions literally stopped for nearly a year because they were not "urgent or emergent" health issues as determined by prison security, health authorities, and community physicians. Compromising care for cardiac, diabetic, neurologic and other patient conditions while directing nearly all human and financial resources to deal with COVID likely affected the longevity of many people with treatable illnesses. I talked to and comforted many inmates' family members who feared their loved ones would die in prison from unaddressed health conditions. Perceived lack of transparency by prison leadership truly worried family members since on-site visitation was eliminated in March 2020, although telephone, video visits and emails still occurred. These communication methods sometimes had a cost to inmates and their families, leading inmates to make outrageous, false claims of them dying from various cancers, Hepatitis C, and COVID. Often-times, inmates played on family sympathy to get deposits made into their prison trust accounts so they could stock up on junk food (e.g., pork rinds, Ramen noodles, honey buns, soft drinks), athletic shoes, and other goods from the Commissary (prison store). Ironically, a percentage of Commissary sales is revenue for the prison system and some contractors. With a few exceptions, food items sold are extremely unhealthy for a prison population with high rates of obesity, hypertension, hyperlipidemia, diabetes and other diagnoses contributed to by poor dietary habits.

In the Fall of 2020 at Coffeewood Correctional Center in Virginia, the warden sent out a memo asking that all family calls regarding healthcare be referred to the warden's office or operations manager. While they did consult with me and our nursing director at times about family concerns, this filtering of information put up an unnecessary wall between the community and medical operations. I believe it added to family mistrust of the system as well.

On a positive note, early in the COVID Pandemic, the HSU posted on the website, VADOC.gov, daily COVID infections for inmates and staff as well as death statistics. This was an admirable action and led to news stories in print and broadcast media that called for early release of medically-vulnerable inmates. Over 2020, the VADOC and HSU also released over 20 revised guidelines for COVID management based on Centers for Disease Control and Prevention (CDC) recommendations to prison and healthcare leaders. This was often overwhelming for security and medical staff, but was a valiant effort to stay current on virus prevention and management.

Nationally, at this time, there were reported shortages of personal protective equipment (PPE) that was vital to keeping health workers safe. Despite a huge stockpile of PPE purchased by VADOC to be proactive, rationing of PPE by prison business office staff and wardens necessitated reuse of disposable masks and gowns on occasion. This practice potentially led to cross-contamination and additional cases of employee and inmate illnesses. As HSA, I often found myself negotiating with the assistant warden and others to get adequate PPE supplies from the stockpile and ordering additional supplies at my employer's expense to fill gaps.

The coronavirus was brought into prisons by security staff, other correctional staff, and in rare cases by healthcare workers. The professed conservative nature of many workers in corrections aligned them with President Donald Trump's early opinion that masks were not needed and COVID-19 was just like the flu. This was a confusing time. Initial conflicting reports from national authorities as to COVID transmission methods resulted in many workers not understanding the need to be masked. These false beliefs led to mandatory masks worn at work, often with only the mouth covered and nose exposed, and no masks after quitting time. Many staff talked about and posted on Facebook their get-togethers with friends after-hours and on weekends to eat, drink and, for some, ultimately become infected.

For all correctional workers, there also was the staffing reality that if they called out when feeling badly, they would be chastised by supervisors. Once COVID test swabs were collected for inmates and staff during "point prevalence" testing, the management focus changed as positive results came in. "If you feel sick, do not come into work," became the daily mantra of the assistant warden at Coffeewood Correctional Center when infection rates were climbing. Temperature check and daily health questionnaire stations were set-up at one or two checkpoints at each prison to catch symptomatic or exposed employees before they entered the facility. Sadly, the infrared thermometers manufactured primarily in China and issued to VADOC prisons were terribly inaccurate. I frequently had a temperature reading two to five degrees lower when on the prison driveway than my reading inside the building lobby only minutes later. These inaccuracies were also commonplace among my co-workers. I strongly advocated for changing the infrared thermometers to temporal or oral thermometers for greater accuracy, but received many excuses for leaving the flawed process in place. Additionally, the majority of the staff cases were asymptomatic (no cough, cold, headaches, loss of taste or smell, or other symptoms) and they were afebrile (fever-free) while still contagious to peers and inmates. The daily health questionnaire, if answered honestly by employees, was the better tool. Unfortunately, fear or ignorance by employees, still resulted in COVID outbreaks within the prisons.

Author Simon Sinek stated this situation well in a post: "When the people have to manage dangers from inside the organization, the organization itself becomes less able to face the dangers from outside" (LinkedIn, 2/19/21).

Chapter 3

Healthcare Behind
the Razor Wire

Introduction

The walled prisons we see in the movies and on TV
dramas are found in parts of Texas and some other
states, but not in the Georgia, Montana, Nevada, New
Mexico, Oklahoma, Tennessee or Virginia facilities
where I have worked. Instead, tall chain link fences
topped with multiple, intertwined strands of razor wire,
often-antiquated surveillance cameras, and correctional
officers equipped with two-way radios, oleoresin
capsicum (OC) spray and handcuffs contain inmates
behind heavy steel doors in housing, dining, education,
medical, vocational, and other areas. Since correctional
officers are trained in weapon use, but unarmed on a
daily basis at the facility levels where I worked, when
serious confrontations or outbursts occurred, specially-
trained, armed "Strike Force" members and, at times,
dogs with handlers could have responded. Generally,
limited movement of inmates keeps confrontations

on the grounds (called the boulevard) to a minimum. Fighting is usually more common in housing units and on recreation yards over gang issues, home-made "mash" alcohol, drugs, unpaid gambling debts, politics or sports rivalry. Gangs including Bloods, Crips, MS-13, White Supremacists and others are carefully monitored, but unpredictable in how they may respond when conflicts arise. Most inmates I have spoken to keep out of the way of aggressors or hang out with buddies for protection. Others seen in our clinics have been severely disfigured from losing fights or attempting to defend themselves. We have sent inmates to hospital emergency departments with concussions, hand fractures, detached eyes, broken jaws, and punctured lungs, among other injuries. During my years working in Virginia, an officer was brutally beaten by an inmate at Sussex Correctional Center, a higher-level prison, when he escorted a nurse on pill call deliveries in a housing unit. After knocking the male officer to the ground, the felon repeated kicked him in the head and yelled to the nurse: "My problem is with him, not you, get the hell out of here." She was traumatized and eventually left correctional nursing. The officer was hospitalized and survived his physical injuries. It is uncertain what became of the violent inmate.

Throughout my years in correctional healthcare, I have seen medical and nursing staff verbally harangued, but never physically-injured by an inmate. I attribute this to the belief that inmates know we are there to help them. In contrast, they associate security staff with outside law enforcement authorities who they blame for being incarcerated. As one warden once quipped, "everyone here swears they're innocent."

Medical Care with Compassion

I do believe that committing a crime requires punishment, but even a criminal deserves humane treatment. As healthcare workers in corrections, my colleagues and I do not need to know the crimes committed by our patients. We are not there to judge them. They have already been judged in a courtroom. Our role is to address their health issues as we would in community clinics. My Christian beliefs guide my concern for friends and enemies alike. In my career I encouraged my staff to live by the Golden Rule and take inmate health issues as seriously as they would the concerns of a family member or friend.

However, many inmates are masters of manipulation and look for weakness in everyone they encounter. Once they hone in on staff they believe can be manipulated, it can result in inappropriate demands for drugs (prescribed and illegal), sexual favors, and other forms of fraternization. Throughout my correctional healthcare years, I have seen nurses, a medication aide, a food services supervisor, and a counselor terminated for fraternization after being observed in sexual relationships (including a prostitution ring using a Texas prison x-ray suite after clinic hours as a sexual meeting place for nurse-inmate intimacy away from security cameras), gift giving, and distributing marijuana and suboxone strips to inmates. One nurse at a prison in Virginia left her long-time boyfriend and moved to West Virginia with an inmate when he was released. She had been in a relationship with him during working hours and resigned before investigators could recommend her termination. She left her significant other in the middle of the night with her school-age children in tow. Another nurse coworker drove the nurse and her family to their new home with the ex-con.

Assistant Warden Tikki Hicks, one of my mentors in Virginia corrections, was known to say: "Kindness is not a weakness; it is a strength." She lived this belief as the #2 in command at Coffeewood Correctional Facility and I saw from her example that firm but fair is an effective leadership style. I also believe I must have a kind heart to lead with integrity. I strived over my years in prison healthcare leadership to be kind to all, but to clearly delineate between being friendly and being friends with co-workers and inmates. Friendships between staff and inmates, as well as staff and other staff, also led to numerous diversions of narcotics and misappropriation of prescription medications. This was reported by some nursing staff with integrity and covered up by others (who ultimately were terminated). Ivan Gilmore, my first warden in Virginia, a former high school stand-out football player, State Trooper and decades-long warden, stressed the importance of "inspect what you expect." That is a leadership trait that is greatly needed in corrections and free world leadership. When we fail to effectively communicate and fail to follow-up, if an employee errs, we both are responsible for the failure.

A Community Standard for All

As discussed previously, inmates in Texas and Virginia, largely because of lawsuits following prison deaths from improper medical care, have legal mandates from the Judiciary to receive all necessary care at no cost if they are indigent or minimal charge if they have money in their trust funds. Legally speaking, "community-level" healthcare is mandated for inmates as wards of the states. It is a sad irony that hard working, law-abiding citizens in our country without insurance or covered by high deductible insurance plans face financial hardships and limited access to care, but inmates receive on-site primary medical care and access to specialists in community hospitals and via telemedicine. Fortunately, expansion of Medicaid in 39 states and the District of Columbia over the past few years has enabled millions of low-income, working Americans to receive the care they deserve. Eleven states have not adopted the Medicaid expansion. These include Alabama, Florida, Georgia, Kansas, Mississippi, North Carolina, South Carolina, Tennessee, Texas, Wisconsin and Wyoming (kff.org, 11/9/22). Medicaid expansion covered inmates in the states where it was approved as well. When inmates agreed to apply for Medicaid and were hospitalized for more than 24 hours for surgery or intensive medical treatment, Medicaid paid the bill. This saved the DOC and the healthcare contractors from paying what would not have been covered by their insurance plan. Ironically, for law-abiding middle-class Americans, individual and family insurance plans on Healthcare.gov (introduced in 2010 as part of the Affordable Care Act or Obamacare) or employer-sponsored plans are cost-prohibitive but the only options available.

Chapter 4

A Healing Environment

While the Virginia DOC is rightfully proud of its healing environment goal and offers educational and behavioral programs to change lives for the better, the primary mission of the Virginia correctional system and other Departments of Corrections is public safety. This is most appropriate, but subject to daily interpretation by wardens, correctional officers and healthcare workers. While one Virginia inmate did walk away from a work camp in 2019 when his officers were not watching, he was rounded up and put in a more secure prison. Overall, prisons nationally are well-contained, safe neighbors and employ hundreds of workers at each facility.

Staff turnover, a shortage of qualified candidates (33% to 75% of positions are unfilled nationally and vary by region) and low pay for correctional officers (average $35,444 in Virginia to $45,000 annually in Nevada) leaves room for future problems. For many, once they are certified as correctional officers, they apply for higher paying positions in county and federal corrections agencies or with police departments. In

Virginia, the average salary for a police officer is $43,869 (ziprecruiter.com), 20% more than a correctional officer earns. With high turnover and vacancy rates, it is not an overstatement to say the inmates are running some of the prisons where there is weak or indecisive leadership and overworked, limited staff.

Most wardens will simply lock-down their prisons when there are too many staff call-outs to safely monitor the inmates. When there is unrest in housing from fights, vandalism, or disobedience of prison policies, lock-downs allow for cooling off and consequences for bad behavior in inmate communities (housing units). This works well in the short-term.

Inmate Economics

However, from my healthcare perspective, overly lengthy lock-downs seen during flu and COVID outbreaks increased inmate tension and anxiety. Since large numbers of inmates in prisons have mental health diagnoses ranging from Attention Deficit Hyperactivity Disorder (ADHD) to bipolar disorder to depression to Post-Traumatic Stress Disorder (PTSD) to schizophrenia, acting out becomes commonplace when inmates are only given one hour to a few hours of time on the recreation yard to breathe fresh air, exercise, and not feel caged in. Additionally, brown bag or Styrofoam container meals during lock-downs replace hot meals and dining hall socialization during the three daily meals.

Food costs are a big factor in prisons. Generally, meals in Virginia prisons cost about $2 per day for each inmate. Labor costs are especially low since limited staff supervise dozens of inmate workers in meal preparation. Despite federal minimum wage laws with a base of $7.25 per hour in most states and ongoing national efforts to raise the minimum wage over time to $15 per hour, Virginia inmates earn less than fifty cents per hour to prepare meals for their peers and staff. In contrast, I was a nursing facility administrator over 20 years ago in North Carolina. Our budgeted food cost was $3.90 per resident per day to feed 100 elderly men and women very healthy, balanced meals. Our staff at the time earned approximately $9 per hour. Prison meals for inmates under the $2 per person budget are high in starch and carbohydrates. Typically, beans are served at least five days per week. Potatoes, white bread, rice and vegetables devoid of nutritional value from overcooking are other mainstays. On rare occasions, meats are served, with "chicken on the bone" or "yard bird" (chicken in the free world) most appreciated by inmates. There is a "common fare" diet option in many prisons originally designed for Jewish and Muslim inmates eating kosher or halal diets. In Virginia prisons, it was considerably healthier for inmates in the beginning, but evolved to be heavily soybean foods that irritated sensitive stomachs.

Staff dining in states offering free meals for employees is considerably more appetizing with chicken, beef, and soup and salad bar in some prisons. Nachos, hot dogs, and sandwiches are served in others. The prisons buy overstock prepackaged soups and desserts, at times frozen before or after expiration dates. Baskin-Robbins ice cream from a year or two after expiration still tastes great!

Prisons have different levels of incarceration based on inmate crime, length of sentence, gang affiliation, and behavior, among other factors. Dormitory housing with single beds and bunkbeds bolted to cement floors are found in lower security level prisons, while single cell and segregation environments are utilized for more violent offenders and those requiring protective custody. Thin, vinyl-covered foam mattresses are definitely uncomfortable and some inmates experience acute and chronic back pain. Day and night, digital surveillance systems provide a means for security officers to watch inmates as they interact, receive medication, get dressed, eat and sleep. This surveillance also alerts officers to altercations as varied as a fist fight to a shank (prison-made knife) thrust in an opponent's chest. Unfortunately, blind spots in prison housing and privacy required in bathrooms leave vulnerable inmates open to aggressors' attacks. Out-of-site spots also are havens for drug dealing, tattooing, gambling and sexual predators. What is not seen can lead to sexual abuse, with young, LGBTI, and mentally ill inmates most vulnerable. In 2003, President George W. Bush signed into federal law the Prison Rape Elimination Act (PREA) to deter sexual assault of prisoners by other inmates and facility staff. Annual PREA education for prison staff reminds workers that there is zero tolerance of sexual assault, sexual abuse, sexual harassment, and sex acts. There is no such thing as consensual sex between a prisoner and another prisoner or prisoner and a prison employee. Sadly, I have served on committees investigating prison rapes and some cases are proven. The mental trauma from being violated is life-altering.

Pain and Disease Management

Pain is one of the most common complaints seen in prison medical clinics. Tylenol, Advil and Mobic are most often given to inmates for pain. Many people in prisons were addicted to prescribed or illegally purchased opioids before incarceration. Others self-medicated with marijuana, heroin, suboxone, fentanyl, methamphetamines, and other substances to numb chronic pain or cope with altered realities. Hundreds of prescribed medications on a drug formulary are also dispensed at pill windows or in dormitories early in the morning and late afternoon for diabetes, hypertension, hyperlipidemia and other chronic illnesses, as well as for acute infections and illnesses. During the COVID Pandemic, to lessen inmate movement, many inmates received the right to keep a 30-day supply of non-narcotic medications in their lockers. This was a good decision that likely increased medication compliance, but some offenders were caught selling their prescriptions to other prisoners. Before and after the Pandemic, "keep on person" medications were given to inmates who agreed to take their health maintenance medications as prescribed. This practice helped many inmates to effectively self-manage high blood pressure, diabetes, asthma and other conditions.

Prison Mercantile

There are some comforts of home in prison life available for inmates with money in their trust funds. Many inmates have personal size TV sets and digital music and game players that they purchase when shopping at the Commissary. Sales of electronics, non-prison-issued tennis shoes, snack foods and other personal items on Commissary generate revenue for both contractors and the DOC. Families and friends of inmates often make regular deposits into trust accounts since few inmates have the means to earn money while incarcerated. When permitted to work, inmates in most states are paid less than fifty cents per hour to scrub toilets, repair air conditioners and heaters, landscape prison grounds, cook inmate and staff meals, work in production facilities for eyeglasses, furniture and clothing, clean staff offices, and act as orderlies in medical clinics. In a few states, inmate jobs are an unpaid privilege. Earnings, along with deposits made by families and attorneys into trust funds managed by prison business office staff, make some personal comforts possible. Commissary purchases are also bartered with other prisoners to pay off gambling debts, avoid life-threatening confrontations with gang members and other hate groups, and get a prison tattoo (with the unexpected consequence of Hepatitis C since prisoner-made tattoo guns and stolen sewing or medical needles are not sterile).

Chapter 5

The Prognosis is Poor

Introduction

In December 2020, I parted ways with Armor Health as HSA at Coffeewood Correctional Center over management differences and health and safety issues that were being ignored by my employer's top leadership.

What I Saw That Made Me Ill

I witnessed patients' lives being put at risk when nurses made medication errors or failed to document administration of medications. Furthermore, outside specialist appointments to see cardiologists and orthopedic surgeons and appointments for Magnetic Resonance Imaging (MRIs) and Computerized Tomography (CT) scans were delayed far longer than the COVID Pandemic's office closures required.

Staff safety was also affected by co-workers leaving new and used insulin syringes, as well as souffle cups and envelopes of medications, on desks. I discovered multiple red bags of infectious waste (blood-soiled linens and used PPE) and discarded disinfectant spray aerosol cans in the hallway of the medical observation unit instead of being locked in a closet for weekly disposal. On another day, I discovered a small oxygen cylinder sitting unsecured in a treatment area that could have become a missile-like projectile if thrown or dropped, or a deadly weapon if used by an inmate to attack another person in the clinic. Still, on another day, three motorized pumice stone tools used for diabetic foot care went missing when a nurse left them outside of a locked storage cabinet. The assistant warden and chief of security were livid and explained to us that the motors would likely be used as part of homemade tattoo guns. Even more concerning were the pumice stones which could be used to file through chain link fences. After many hours of searching by correctional officers and investigators, the tools remained unfound.

I held the director of nursing accountable for her nurses' performance, but she treated my concerns as minor and, as a result, the behavior of some of her direct reports worsened. Finally, one weekend when I reached out to her for advice on whom to contact when there was an unexpected call-out (and the on-call nurse claimed she was unaware of being on call) she resigned via a text message, saying she was "done". I immediately accepted her 30-day notice. However, after being urged by the warden and a few co-workers to ask her to stay, I gave her the opportunity to rescind the resignation because I truly wanted her to work with me on the team's performance improvement. However, she had other plans. Instead of supporting the necessary disciplinary actions and greater staff accountability, the nursing director reached out to Armor-Virginia leadership in Richmond and fabricated an account of my "yelling at staff" and "delegating all my work to others" to deflect from her lack of nursing oversight. I assume she suggested I had created a hostile work environment. Since Armor-Virginia (at the time) was led by a president who was an attorney, the nursing director created doubt and fear of employment litigation. She played both of us to her advantage.

The truth regarding my "yelling at the staff" was that I raised my voice one time towards an inmate and later apologized to him. I never raised my voice to anyone on the staff. Also, my average work week was over 50 hours because of all the tasks I needed to complete. Her average work week was barely 40 hours; so, hours worked were indisputable.

Twenty-two months earlier, I had hired this director of nursing in her mid-20's even though she lacked correctional experience. She had good hospital experience and I believe strongly in offering jobs to people seeking new opportunities. She was eager to learn a new field and had a fascination with forensic medicine. To help her be successful, I scheduled the retired former director of nursing, an outstanding RN, to mentor her. This was a great investment in the new director. Sadly, when she was put to the test and tough action was needed, she attacked my character instead of dealing with the problems. On December 3, 2020 I had a meeting with Armor-Virginia's vice president of nursing in person and the Armor-Virginia president on speakerphone. I was not allowed to share my side of the story. The nursing director's indictment of my character was simply accepted as fact. When I resigned, I was asked to sign a lengthy separation agreement that would silence me personally and shield me from suing

Armor in return for a month's severance pay. Since I received the document within minutes via email, I can only surmise that I was not the first employee to be separated in this manner. As I marked my thirty-fourth year as a healthcare professional in 2020, it was clear to me that it was time to move on and mentor others who share my ethical values. My integrity is priceless and I am fully transparent in my relationships with staff and patients alike.

I began my Virginia correctional career with MedikoPC at Coffeewood, then joined VADOC at Fluvanna Correctional Center for Women (FCCW), and finally Armor to lead healthcare for Greensville Correctional Center, the largest male prison in Virginia. When Armor abruptly reassigned me back to Coffeewood, my career unexpectedly came full circle. Since my wife and I owned a home over two hours from Greensville Correctional, we sold our house and planned to move to Petersburg, VA. On the week of our property's closing, I had a three-month performance evaluation by Armor's regional nurse manager. I was praised for the excellent staff I recruited and told how much the team liked me. As with most reviews, I was also offered some opportunities for improvement. Then a bombshell exploded: the final paragraph of the evaluation abruptly reassigned me back to Coffeewood, the smaller male facility where I previously worked under MedikoPC, a regional competitor to Armor. VADOC and MedikoPC parted ways and their contracts for Coffeewood and Augusta Correctional Centers were awarded to Armor effective July 1, 2020. Armor hired all but one nurse who was on worker's comp, the HSA who had replaced me when I left to join VADOC, and the medical director.

The departing HSA and I spoke on two occasions and he warned me that the director of nursing "threw him under the bus" and I should be careful. His warning proved true.

When COVID Hit Home

During my quarter of a year at Greensville in 2020, I contracted the coronavirus. My office in the building housing the prison infirmary was a "Red Zone," a designation denoting all patients were diagnosed with COVID and were being carefully monitored for temperature, oxygen level, blood pressure and worsening disease complications. Many suffered a loss of taste and smell. Others experienced fevers of 100.4 or higher, leading to dehydration and other health issues. Severe headaches were common but easily treated. Oxygen levels under 94% and breathing difficulties often led to hospitalizations to treat pneumonia and other lung infections. For some with histories of Chronic Obstructive Pulmonary Disease (COPD), ventilators were employed to artificially breathe for the hospitalized inmates. Many of the inmates at the Greensville Infirmary were high risk: older, ethnic minorities, diabetic, co-morbidities of hypertension or cancer, or on dialysis. While my co-workers and I wore masks and appropriate PPE when in patient care areas, the recirculation of air conditioning most likely spread the virus from patient zones into offices. There were 10 medically-designed, reverse flow isolation rooms at the Greensville Infirmary that did not recirculate air beyond their doors, but the large number of COVID+ inmates spilled over into open air wards and infected others. The Greensville medical director, infection control nurse and caregiving staff worked valiantly to monitor inmates' health. Losses could have been far-greater if this team had not worked so well together.

As a consequence of my work life at Greensville, I became an asymptomatic (symptom-free) COVID+ patient and unknowingly infected my wife and my mother-in-law, who were hospitalized for three days and nearly a month respectively. My wife was treated for pneumonia and was on low levels of supplemental oxygen when discharged from a Charlottesville, VA hospital with a rolling e-cylinder oxygen tank in tow. She also developed excessively high ferritin (iron) levels in her blood and a deep vein thrombosis (DVT) in her left leg that required months of taking Eliquis, an expensive blood-thinning medication that has unsettling side effects. My mother-in-law, an insulin-dependent diabetic, was on a ventilator. During her hospitalization, poor care by a nurse at a Maryland hospital starting an IV led to a severe infection that required a skin graft to her arm and ongoing hand therapy. A normally active woman at age 76, unfortunately she will likely never fully regain use of one hand as a result of the injury that could have been avoided or caught earlier (while still treatable). Her driving skills were affected and she could not fully grip items with one hand.

I never expected my prison work to impact my family as it did and my employer showed little concern for my family's plight. As a consolation prize for the sudden move from Greensville to Coffeewood, I was given one week of paid time off. My wife and I took a trip to the Outer Banks in North Carolina, unaware that I had an asymptomatic case of COVID. Shortly after we returned from vacation, I developed a high fever and tested positive for the virus. Since we sold our home and were searching for a house to buy, we stayed first at two Airbnb homes, then isolated ourselves in two hotel rooms at our expense. When the dust settled, the total financial cost to my family for my service as an Armor administrator was considerable. The emotional cost cannot be computed. By 2022, Armor lost their Virginia contracts.

Chapter 6

Virginia Women's Prison Care Was Newsworthy

Introduction

Fluvanna Correctional Center for Women (FCCW) is the largest women's prison in Virginia and is home to approximately 1200 level three felons as well as women with severe mental illness underlying their criminal activity. FCCW was designed with a 78,000 sq. ft. medical facility on site. Services for inmates include a primary care clinic that operates Monday-Friday with six staff and locum (temporary agency) medical doctors and nurse practitioners seeing up to 100 patients a day for acute and chronic conditions. A 26-bed infirmary and medical observation unit are staffed by registered nurses, licensed professional nurses and certified nurse aides 24/7. An acute mental health unit is also on site. Other services include on-site dental, physical therapy, mental healthcare, laboratory, dialysis, optometry and podiatry. A radiology suite provides general x-rays, ultrasounds, fibroscans for Hepatitis C assessment, and mammograms. Pharmacy services are provided up to four times daily by LPNs with pill carts in offender housing and pill windows. Many medications are available as Keep On Person (KOP) in 30-day blister packs for self-administration All of these resources would lead one to believe the health care was exceptional. In truth, failures in the care delivery system resulted in unwanted attention by the press and the courts.

Medical Drama in The Women's Prison

When FCCW's healthcare services were operated by Armor Health, the unexpected deaths of three women led to the court case Scott et al v. Clarke et al and subsequent judicial oversight. Additionally, the facility's healthcare services were transitioned from Armor to the VADOC. In November 2019, I left Coffeewood Correctional Center and MedikoPC and was hired by the VADOC HSU director to become the healthcare program manager at FCCW. My charge was to work with the medical director and warden to set quality improvement processes in place and get the prison out from under the lawsuit. I was excited to take on the challenge and believed I could make a difference. My interview panel included the chief nurse for VADOC, a nurse manager reporting to her, and a former warden/current VADOC contract administrator. Cindy Morgan, a nurse practitioner and former HSA at Dillwyn Correctional Center I greatly respected, was acting director of nursing, so I was very optimistic we could make the needed systemic changes to correct the issues noted in the lawsuit.

Before I accepted the position at FCCW, I was warned by colleagues that "the prisoners run the prison and will soon be getting a swimming pool," "women inmates are very needy," "the women are all crazy," "nobody wants to work at FCCW because the nurses eat their young," and "it's not safe to work there because they are dangerously short of correctional officers." What I found was an adversarial relationship between many on the medical staff and the inmates. The fact that a court monitor regularly checked on quality of care did result in more accessible care for these inmates, but whether or not it was higher quality of care is debatable. To use a sports analogy, while physicians and nurse practitioners were the quarterbacks on the healthcare football team and determined the plays (diagnoses and treatments), the nurses and other staff ran the ball (direct care). At FCCW, the team had record numbers of fumbles. Unlike football, healthcare fumbles can have deadly consequences.

As for the warnings I received, the inmates never did get a swimming pool. They did get some preferential treatment, however, by working the system and routinely threatening more lawsuits. Instead of requesting doctor appointments as male prisoners were required to do, many FCCW inmates used the emergency grievance written process for minor health issues. In these reportedly urgent cases, VADOC policy requires the patient to be evaluated or treated by a clinician within eight hours, when normal sick call appointments took three days or more to be seen. This was often a poor use of clinic resources but lessened complaints to the monitor—a prominent correctional physician from Pennsylvania— or the Legal Aid Justice Center in Charlottesville, VA that had continued to advocate for them after the court decision.

In my work with both female and male inmates, I find that women inmates have more health issues and often require more time from health providers due to preventative care like pap smears and breast exams, as well as recurrent health concerns like urinary tract infections. However, the men in prisons can also be drama queens. Some of the toughest men I have met with violent rap sheets, top-to-bottom tattoos, and gang affiliations fear getting a flu shot or having blood drawn. At times, they claim to be dying over ingrown toenails, hemorrhoids and constipation.

Faking seizures to get medical attention or a brief respite from prison housing is commonplace in prisons for both sexes. This can make treating real seizures challenging. There is a simple "diagnostic tool" for seizures I learned from prison nurses. When the "seizing" patient lays on the ground in a restful moment, the nurse lifts the patient's arm high above his or her head. She then drops it. The patient with a true seizure gets a slap in their face and the loss of consciousness from a seizure or another cause is confirmed. The faker stops their arm before getting slapped. It really works. Also, when a true seizure occurs, it is common for the patient to defecate or urinate in their pants, so a "smell test" can be part of the diagnostic drill. When patients have histories of extensive illegal drug use, many develop seizure disorders that can be prevented or lessened in intensity with medications used to treat epilepsy.

Prisoner Mental Health Issues

As for the sanity of the inmates at FCCW, the sheer number of women on psychiatric medications, the large staff of mental health workers employed, and the dedicated mental health unit do give credence to the claim of many mentally ill women living there. I was advised by a psychiatrist who had previously worked at FCCW that 75% of these inmates had a mental health diagnosis and were on psychiatric medications. Others were drug abusers; and their long-term drug use had affected thinking processes, led to impulsivity, and resulted in health issues from damaged hearts to kidney and liver disorders. In addition, many were victims of domestic abuse by male or female companions.

Many in our society are quick to shy away from discussing mental illness and most communities lack adequate mental health services for the uninsured. With these realities in society, women with bipolar disorder, schizophrenia, and other mental illnesses often act erratically and end up getting arrested, convicted and incarcerated. Sadly, many of these women lacked clear thinking (and likely were unmedicated) in their communities and wound up in mentally- or physically-abusive homes. Abuse led to further dysfunction such as job loss, homelessness, isolation, and criminal acts ranging from shoplifting to selling drugs to striking back and injuring or killing spousal abusers. If mental illness in the "free world" was treated with the same level of care that we give to physical illnesses like diabetes and hypertension, the number of incarcerated people would surely decrease. The answer does not simply lie with availability of prescriptions. A holistic approach must include counseling, education, housing assistance, and ongoing support systems in the public before the mentally ill commit crimes and become wards of the State.

Medical Staffing Shortages

As for the statement that "nobody wants to work at FCCW (Medical) because the nurses eat their young," I definitely witnessed overt prejudice by two Caucasian nurse managers toward African-American co-workers and one case of ongoing discrimination by one African-American support staff supervisor towards an older Caucasian employee. Cliques were present in specific nursing units and some staff refused to work where needed outside of their comfort zones—even when offered the necessary training. The attitude by many entrenched staff and agency nurses towards me and my acting director of nursing was "you need me more than I need you." That view did not bode well for teamwork.

When interviewing new staff, I shared my belief that correctional nursing is not for everyone, but it is a great place for those interested in public health. I also shared that they would experience a learning opportunity and see unusual illnesses. It was their opportunity to use their education and experience to fully assess patients and save lives. Had all the nursing leadership team I inherited shared my beliefs, we could have developed a great group of empathetic nurses. Sadly, there was so much negativity and sense of entitlement by staff and agency nurses at FCCW that the idea of being kind to and shepherding new nurses was not going to occur. The turnover of new staff continued. Even some highly-paid agency nurses from North Carolina and West Virginia did not renew contracts because they never felt welcomed or supported. "It's not only about the Benjamins," aptly quipped one nurse.

As for the claim "it's not safe to work there because they are dangerously short of correctional officers," this rang true when I learned that a sergeant I had worked with and respected at Coffeewood had accepted a promotion to lieutenant at FCCW, but quickly returned back to his former prison "because he did not feel safe with the poor staffing at FCCW." A year earlier at Coffeewood, this experienced officer who stands nearly 6'5" and is built like a football linebacker demonstrated his fearlessness. With very little support from other staff, he stopped a riot of almost 25 inmates that spilled out from a dining hall onto the boulevard by tackling the leader of the uprising and sitting on him until other officers responded. The warden did not approve of his tactic, but all of us co-workers felt a little bit safer because of his actions.

I was very mindful of my surroundings when walking on the FCCW campus, but I definitely saw how short staffed the prison was and worried about my team's safety. Lockdowns of housing units and limited inmate movement was the warden's response to being short staffed and this was comforting to staff, but stressful for inmates.

When I arrived, FCCW Medical was being operated with 70% of the staff coming from contracted nursing staffing agencies at pay rates as high as 50% to 100% higher than the 30% who were employed directly by the Commonwealth. The reality at FCCW was their reputation was so bad that most nurses in the area with any other viable career options would not work there.

Since I had changed community perceptions in past jobs by hiring quality clinicians and building strong teams, I thought I could change that perception, attract nurses that shared my vision, and save taxpayers millions of dollars in unnecessary labor costs. There was an unhealthy co-dependency by some nurse managers with the two contracted staffing agencies providing the majority of staff and rumors quickly spread that I was going to "get rid of all agency nurses." I tried to clarify my intention in a staff meeting by explaining that there will always be some agency staff in this size facility, but the numbers need to be flipped. My goal was to offer jobs as State employees to all agency staff at the end of their contracts. In a year, I hoped to have 70% to 80% employed by VADOC and 20% to 30% from agencies. Fear of the unknown frightens many of us, but some of the nursing managers responded poorly to my leadership efforts. Cindy Morgan and I brought in some new staff nurses and converted a few agency nurses to staff positions, but it was like we were swimming upstream against rapids.

Despite massive recruitment efforts, when I tried to hire a new director of nursing to give Cindy an opportunity to return to her nurse practitioner role at other prisons, no qualified candidates were willing to join a facility with legal problems and a community image of "nurses eating their young." Three internal candidates were interviewed twice by a panel and none were recommended for hire. In a compromise of necessity, one internal nurse manager who had been fired from a hospital for violating an emergency room policy with no remorse, but was a hard worker at FCCW, was named the interim director of nursing. The interview panel believed her clinical skills were solid, but her brash personality and lack of remorse over the hospital policy violation were troublesome. I needed support from VADOC Security and Health Services leadership to bring about real change. The assistant director of health services in Richmond fought valiantly for me to institute much needed changes, but he stood alone.

My Last Days at FCCW

Unfortunately, I was not able to meet the medical director, warden, or most of the nursing staff prior to my hire. For nearly one month I was stationed in Richmond at the VADOC headquarters, where I was briefed on the lawsuit and attended operational meetings. During that month, the HSU assistant director, staff recruiter and I developed an organizational chart that illustrated my leadership responsibilities and operational areas. Unfortunately, once I arrived at FCCW this plan proved short lived as I dug in to identify health and safety issues, address a nurse manager's falsification of time records, and other concerns that shined a bright light on the current operational realities at FCCW. Security leadership at VADOC did not want to hear about other issues at FCCW, and I later learned that I was not the first to try to fix a broken prison healthcare system. My predecessor, a nurse with many years in the VADOC, could not see eye-to-eye with the warden and was reassigned to VADOC headquarters. I am a high energy healthcare administrator with a strong sense of ethics, so I cannot just ignore risky healthcare practices, waste taxpayer dollars, and accept dysfunctional teams.

In well-functioning healthcare systems, my traits are admired. At FCCW, sadly, that was not the case.

When I had the opportunity to meet the medical director, I was quite impressed with his academic credentials. He had worked at the Mayo Clinic prior to joining the University of Virginia (UVA). He was viewed by VADOC leaders as the physician champion to deliver them from the lawsuit—at any cost. His VADOC annual salary of $325,000 was higher than his peers and other State physicians with greater leadership responsibilities. He also continued to see patients at UVA Healthcare and was an associate professor earning $240,000 prior to joining VADOC. Comparatively, the VADOC chief medical director over all Virginia prisons earned $240,778, VADOC Director Harold Clarke earned $189,112, and Virginia Governor and Pediatric Neurologist Ralph Northam earned $175,000 according to 2019 published salaries (https://www.bizjournals.com/washington/news/2019/10/04/public-paychecks-who-earns-the-most-on-virginias.html).

The warden had a love-hate relationship with the medical director, and never introduced me to his leadership team. He overstepped his operational boundaries by micromanaging medical staff without respect for healthcare chain of command, and told me he should have been consulted before I was hired. His mistrust of the VADOC HSU leadership led him to accuse me on several occasions of spying on his operation and calling VADOC leadership in Richmond to "throw him under the bus." When I was hired at VADOC, I reported to the assistant director of the HSU and he and I discussed operational issues and strategies, but I never bad mouthed the warden's actions.

As a professional, when I have differences with co-workers, I talk to them directly and usually have success finding common ground. Had the warden given me an opportunity for us to get to know one another, we could have made his prison healthcare program less likely to face future litigation. What ultimately occurred was my activist presence was unwanted by the medical director and warden. The VADOC leadership eventually made major changes to the organizational chart we created and stripped me of all direct report relationships expect for one minor area. The medical director was given back all direct reporting relationships under the guise that "was what the court expected." I was called to VADOC headquarters by the HSU director in late-February 2020 and informed that "I was not a good fit with the warden and medical director." I was allowed to resign when faced with termination and within a month was hired by Armor Health to lead the medical unit at the Greensville Correctional Center, the largest male prison in Virginia.

As fate would have it, the FCCW warden was transferred to Greensville Correctional Center as one of several wardens shortly after Armor hired me to work there. One of his female FCCW assistant wardens, who I greatly respected for her insights and effective communication, was promoted to his senior warden position. As detailed earlier, within three months, I was sent by Armor back to the first prison I worked at in Virginia, Coffeewood Correctional Center. Armor's leadership said "they wanted to avoid any possible conflict with the warden." It was the warden's issue with trust, not mine, but the transfer was non-negotiable.

Chapter 7

Yes, You're Going to Die

Introduction

In my first book, *Extraordinary Encounters in an Ordinary Life,* I shared a joke that has some truth in it. What does MD mean? Major Deity? Medical Doctor? A combination of both? In the case of some of the prison doctors I worked with across the country, the God complex is no laughing matter. These doctors literally have life and death in their hands.

At the beginning of my corrections career, when I worked for the University of Texas Medical Branch Correctional Managed Care (UTMB-Galveston) from 2002 to 2004, I was the practice manager at L.V. Hightower (Men's) Unit and Henley (Women's) State Jail in Dayton, Texas, one hour north of Houston. I then transferred to Dallas where I led healthcare services for the five Dallas County Jails populated by men and women, and Hutchins State Jail, a male facility.

Prison Physicians

The doctors on-site were primarily end-of-career physicians in their 60's through late-70's with a lifetime of experience. Younger Physician Assistants (PAs) and Nurse Practitioners (NPs) also treated patients and were extremely current with modern medicine. Supporting these clinicians was a pioneering telemedicine program that connected our staff with leading academic medical specialists who broadcasted from a state-of-the-art studio at UTMB in Galveston, TX. Orthopedic surgeons, infectious disease specialists, cardiologists, dermatologists and others shared their expertise with primary care doctors on-site at correctional facilities throughout Texas. They saved many lives and considerable taxpayer dollars by avoiding costly, labor-intensive transports from prisons around the Lone Star State to the TDCJ UTMB Hospital in Galveston. Clinicians inside prison and jail clinics were walked through casting broken bones, shared abnormal electrocardiograms (EKGs) and heart anomalies by connecting a stethoscope that transmitted real-time heartbeats, and zoomed in on suspicious wounds and moles to determine proper treatment. I joined the doctors on many of these telemedicine sessions that, 20 years later, are now commonplace in both correctional facilities and throughout the free world. In fact, the COVID Pandemic inspired greater use of telemedicine throughout the world as social distancing and infection control concerns kept face-to-face medical and mental health visits at a minimum. In my years working in Virginia prisons (2017 to 2020), we used telemedicine for psychiatry, hepatology and infectious diseases. Other specialty services were available and used at other prisons. Virginia Commonwealth University/ Medical College of Virginia and the University of Virginia provided these services to Virginia prisoners. In the COVID-era, telemedicine truly was a life-saver as clinics that normally saw inmates closed for many months and only "urgent and emergent" cases were sent to the ER at area hospitals. As a result of the Pandemic and technological advances, many private practice physicians today have become telehealth practitioners for incarcerated populations and the free world, especially in rural, underserved areas.

American author and humorist Mark Twain wrote, "Truth is stranger than fiction, but it is because fiction is obliged to stick to possibilities; truth isn't." TV shows from *M*A*S*H* to *ER* to *The Good Doctor,* have brought viewers inside battlefield hospitals, emergency departments and research hospitals. The movie *One Flew Over the Cuckoo's Nest* took us inside a mental hospital. We have laughed, cried and closed our eyes in disbelief or horror as we tuned in to these fictitious accounts of healthcare. With my hat's off to Mr. Twain, welcome to my years spent in prison medicine. Unlike the TV and movie plots, these stories are real.

The correctional doctors I worked with were quite colorful and their stories, like those penned in Hollywood, can bring out positive and negative emotions. The first doctor I worked with in Texas prisons shortly after the beginning of the twenty-first century was a kind man with a highly unusual background for a prison physician. He was a pathologist for many years, schooled in laboratory examination of samples of body tissue for diagnostic and forensic purposes. He reinvented himself in his 50's to provide primary care in a men's prison.

He was caring, extremely introverted, soft-spoken, and not very sociable. Rarely did he make eye contact with his patients or co-workers, but he did earn our staff's respect. Another correctional physician I worked with was both a doctor and a lawyer. This seemed like a good combination for the five jails we served in Dallas, including one Immigration and Customs Enforcement (ICE) facility that contained multiple chain link cages housing illegal aliens facing deportation.

Mental healthcare at the Dallas County Jails was led by an end-of-career psychiatrist who found me to be overly punitive with one of his male psychiatric PAs, an event that caused conflict in our professional relationship. When the PA was caught by a co-worker watching adult porn on his desktop computer, I had the Dallas County Sheriff's staff investigate his search history and this proved not to be an isolated incident. When I wrote a disciplinary counseling of the employee for the psychiatrist to review and present, I requested psychological counseling and a suspension or termination (to be determined by his supervisor). The psychiatrist supervisor, in turn, defended the PA for a "very normal activity by many men." Since the employee did not view "child porn" his action was deemed not "deviant behavior and required no therapy." The only issue the supervisor agreed to was improper use of a work computer. As practice manager, I disciplined the PA in writing, suspended him for three days, and warned him that future misuse of State computers would have more serious ramifications. It was deeply disturbing to me that the psychiatrist failed to see how the PA's behavior could affect his clinical judgement when counseling sex offenders and other convicted men.

Forgetful Rescuer

Perhaps the most memorable physician I worked with in the TDCJ was a cardiologist in his late-70's. He was a larger-than-life man, standing a few inches taller than my 6'3" frame, and easily weighing over 350 pounds. He had a full head of wavy white hair, a bushy mustache, and looked like a Texas-size model for an American Medical Association brochure or an actor for a remake of the *Marcus Welby, MD* television show of my childhood. Quite distinguished, he always wore his lab coat with stethoscope and prescription reference guide in the pocket. However, looks can be deceiving. He frequently got confused during his shifts. He forgot how to log in to his computer nearly every day and I helped him as often as I could. He would wander around the clinic, apparently with no destination in mind, until steered back into an exam room by a nurse or other co-worker. One of his PAs followed up on the medications he electronically prescribed to ensure the correct drugs were ordered. Then, one day, an inmate in the clinic collapsed from a massive heart attack in front of the doctor. Within seconds the doctor dropped to the floor and began chest compressions on the man. A nurse called 911 and the doctor kept working on the patient with great intensity and clinical competency until he was relieved by a Dallas paramedic. The patient was taken to the hospital and had multiple bypass surgery. He lived to see another day thanks to the instincts of our doctor. Sadly, when I and another staff member talked to the doctor the next workday, the doctor had no memory of this happening.

Thirteen years later, I found similar stories in Virginia. Perhaps my most frustrating interactions with prison doctors involved a former orthopedic surgeon in his mid-70's. He shared with me that he had no hobbies or outside interests, was bored in retirement, and decided to leave his arranged-marriage wife of 50 years at their home in a neighboring state three days a week to stay at a two-star hotel near the prison and work as a primary care physician. Born and educated in India, this Sikh doctor frequently argued with inmates. Poised behind his desk, he visually scanned medical records and talked at the male patients rather than with them. Rarely did he physically examine patients and his bedside manner showed total lack of caring. Over the time we worked together, I responded to hundreds of complaints called informal grievances from inmates about him documenting his indifference to their well-being and callous attitude as "cruel and unusual punishment" and begging me to let them see the other doctor in our clinic. Most disturbing to our patients was when he told them they had an illness and they asked about the seriousness by saying "Can I die from this?" They were told, "We're all going to die."

A Second Opinion Saves the Day

If his lack of empathy was not disturbing enough, his lack of primary care training resulted in misdiagnosing a brain tumor in a man in his early-40's who had debilitating headaches along with a loss of mobility. He also likely shortened the life of a man in his 50's who the doctor kept incorrectly treating for hemorrhoids over many months as undiagnosed pancreatic cancer was spreading. Fortunately for the inmates, we had another doctor who provided medical care two days a week. At this time, a male general practitioner in his 50's was also assigned to our clinic. While he only completed four years of medical school in Mexico and did not have residency training in any specialty, he had an inquisitive mind and empathy for his patients. I took both of these patients' charts to him one day and expressed my fear that the more senior doctor was missing something. At first, the doctor did not want to step on his peer's toes and question his diagnoses and treatments. He argued that I was setting a dangerous precedent by giving the inmates decision-making power over who treats them, but agreed to review the charts. After he did, we scheduled both inmates to be physically examined. The doctor, after taking a thorough medical history and performing a hands-on exam, made urgent referrals for a CT scan to find the underlying cause of the headaches and change in function. He also referred the other man to a colorectal surgeon. When results came back, the brain tumor had been detected, was extremely large and required neurosurgery within days or, in the words of the neurosurgeon, the patient would die. This inmate was due for release from prison the week he was properly diagnosed. Despite his protests, I asked the warden to hold him for a few more weeks so he could get the brain surgery while he had State-paid insurance. The warden agreed that this was best and arranged to hold him for up to one month beyond his release date. Thankfully, he was able to get the surgery and return home to his two young sons. He was angry with us for keeping him incarcerated beyond his sentence, but it was the right decision.

The cancer patient was justifiably angry at the primary doctor and his prognosis was dire. He agreed to undergo cancer treatment at a nearby hospital and this prolonged his life for at least two years, but it was an uncomfortable existence filled with "chemo brain" confusion, weakness, nausea, vomiting and a reality that he would not likely live to see freedom when his scheduled release date came in a few years. He and I talked often and he met with our mental health staff as well, but he knew that he was misdiagnosed and the anger he felt was justified. He threatened to sue for malpractice as did other inmates. The only comfort I truly could offer him was joining one of the prison staff and his oncologist in writing to the Virginia Parole Board seeking early release on medical grounds, which unfortunately proved unsuccessful.

Ignored Symptoms

I believe the final straw for me in my relationship with the senior doctor was when a Chinese-American inmate in his 50's developed body tremors so great that he could barely feed himself without flinging food off his spork (forks are not allowed in Virginia prison inmate dining halls). I had worked in physical rehabilitation, nursing home administration, and with neurologists while at the National Multiple Sclerosis Society, and saw many cases of Parkinson's and other neurologic conditions. I was convinced that Parkinson's was causing the inmate's constant shaking and twitching. He was also malnourished and needed a cane or walker to assist him in safely walking across prison grounds. I scheduled him to see the older doctor because I thought his earlier career as an orthopedic surgeon might be helpful. The inmate was a mechanical engineer before his conviction for a sex crime and used the prison library to conduct extensive research on his symptoms and possible treatments. His illegal activity was disgusting, but I believed he still deserved humane treatment as a human being incarcerated for many years for his crime. After sharing my thoughts with the doctor about this looking like Parkinson's cases I have seen in the past, he rudely reminded me that I was not a doctor but agreed to assess him.

Better late than never, after 9 months, the inmate was sent to a neurologist at Virginia Commonwealth University in Richmond and diagnosed with Parkinson's as I had suspected. The medications prescribed by the neurologist required some tweaking, but the physical changes were remarkable. He also ordered Ensure and an extra portion of food each day. One year after seeing the neurologist, the patient was well-nourished, had only minor uncontrolled movements, and walked confidently with a cane. He was appreciative for my advocacy, but later upset that I agreed with another doctor that he no longer needed Ensure. For this indigent inmate who was disowned by his family and had no funds for Commissary, a chocolate Ensure was a real treat.

I was greatly troubled by the poor care provided by our most senior doctor and I took time one morning to share my concerns with him. He had on numerous occasions reminded me and outspoken nursing staff that we were not doctors, so I was uncertain as to what I could achieve. He encapsulated his thoughts to me in one sentence: "Mr. Miller, medicine is an inexact science."

Angel of Mercy

Months later, I talked with the chief operating officer at MedikoPC, our employer, and he agreed with me to exercise a 30-day termination clause and replace the uncaring clinician with a more appropriate one. The doctor who properly treated the two patients with the brain tumor and cancer was reassigned to another correctional facility before this termination occurred. I recruited a petite, kind, highly-competent female internal medicine physician whose husband had worked for me as a locums (agency) doctor when our senior doctor took a month-long trip overseas. Both physicians had worked together at an urgent care clinic in Northern Virginia prior to retirement. As a result of the staffing change, the inmates and our staff saw a night and day difference in quality of care. She practiced by getting to know her patients by name, conservatively prescribed medications, and was hands-on in her patient care. Ironically, the senior doctor who was terminated by MedikoPC was quickly hired by Armor Health to practice at other prisons. And as Armor took over contracts from MedikoPC, as fate would have it, he and I were reassigned to work together once again at Coffeewood Correctional Center. He did resign a short time later as COVID cases starting growing at the prison. As he was 76-years-old with health issues of his own, I can only assume he listened to his family and decided it was finally time to retire.

Pain Mismanagement

It can be difficult to treat inmates because many were drug abusers and do not respond to over-the-counter pain medications since the illegal drugs they took in the community damaged their nervous systems. Others are drug seeking and are influenced by their peers to demand medications they see on TV or received on the "streets." One inmate who killed a friend and nearly died himself in an auto accident while driving under the influence had intractable pain from the injuries he incurred in the wreck and from over a dozen surgeries he reportedly had to repair his injured body. He was on multiple pain medications and as VADOC reduced the number of medications on the prison formulary, he could no longer receive the specific medication he craved. When MedikoPC was the contractor at Coffeewood and the senior physician was still there, the inmate threatened to "hang him by his turban." I stood alongside the doctor in the exam room at future appointments and met with the inmate often to keep him as calm as possible, but there was an ongoing hate-hate relationship that did not improve no matter what I tried to do. The doctor did file internal charges against the man for threatening violence and his penalty was loss of Commissary for 20 days.

Abuse of Compassion

Towards the end of my first leadership position at Coffeewood, before I joined VADOC at FCCW, MedikoPC CEO Dr. Kaveh Ofogh appointed a physician in his 40's to be our medical director three days per week as the senior doctor had worked before him. Dr. Ofogh also later appointed him as corporate medical director. The new MD was a gregarious fellow with boundless energy and a huge heart. Unfortunately, in correctional medicine, being outwardly kind can lead to clinicians being manipulated by inmates. The good doctor was a strong clinician but in trying so hard to have satisfied patients, he frustrated and alienated nursing staff. He also prescribed medications and medical supplies after being convinced by inmates that they needed them. When compared to other prisons, the Coffeewood medical director ordered four times the number of custom-cast orthotic inserts for boots and tennis shoes that cost over $200 per pair. The Commonwealth of Virginia purchases insurance for incarcerated men and women, but much of the cost is borne by medical contractors like MedikoPC and Armor through "full risk" contracts and taxpayers who ultimately pay for the insurance premiums and contracts in the millions of dollars with MedikoPC, Armor and GEO. In most healthcare organizations, there is a system of checks and balances called utilization management that requires a second, external physician to approve prescriptions that are not on a strict drug formulary and costly diagnostic tests (CT scans, MRIs, Positive Emission Tomography (PET) scans, etc.) ordered by another clinician. When MedikoPC appointed this doctor as corporate and Coffeewood medical director, there was no external review or approval process. Even though I respected this doctor as a strong clinician, I strongly challenged this unusual lack of oversight. I was told by MedikoPC leadership to let it go. The inmate with chronic pain from a deadly auto accident discussed earlier had lobbied hard for better pain management and was prescribed multiple medications and sent to outside pain management specialists by Coffeewood's medical director, only to have most of the medications rescinded cold turkey by Armor's returning senior doctor—once again angering the inmate.

Chapter 8

On the Road in
Correctional Care

Introduction

Joining CoreCivic in the Spring of 2021 as HSA at Coffee Correctional Center in rural South Georgia was an opportunity to be a leader in a correctional company that had strong ethics. The publicly-traded company based in Brentwood, TN was formerly known as Correctional Corporation of America (CCA) and stresses to their employees in 30 states the Be-8 principles. They are:

1) Be Aware
2) Be Respectful
3) Be Communicative
4) Be A Good Decision Maker
5) Be Humble
6) Be Positive
7) Be A Situational Leader
8) Be An Active Participant.

After nearly a year at Coffee Correctional, I was promoted to a role where I would have a greater impact on developing other administrators and improving patient care. In my traveling role as a Surge HSA, I met many dedicated correctional officers in second careers following military service, and medical and support staff with experience ranging from first career after high school or community college to over 20 years of correctional service. Women employees outnumbered men in many prison positions, so interpersonal communication to de-escalate angry inmates clearly was the most appropriate daily strategy rather than using brute force or OC spray. Some correctional officers clearly got caught up in the heat of the moment and yelled curse words in response to inmate taunts. Oftentimes, female officers disrespected by male inmates gave what I call the "Mama talk." They would firmly and often loudly say: "I know you have a Mama. You may have a sister or a daughter too. Would you talk to them like that?" In most cases, the inmates apologized and the message was received.

Illegal drugs, cellphones, and hand-crafted weapons were the most common contraband found in prisons where I have worked. This report from a New Mexico prison in the Summer of 2022 demonstrated how community members threw drugs over prison fences in hopes of reaching friends or family members who are incarcerated.

"Vehicle Patrol Officer saw a black car leaving the area of the facility fence near Truck Stop. Upon search of the area, I saw a stainless steel-like mug wrapped in duct tape outside 800 Bravo. I secured the mug. Interior and exterior window checks were conducted in all cells in 700 and 800. No windows were broken.

The following illegal substances were found inside the mug: 306 unopened Buprenorphine (Suboxone), 193 open Buprenorphine (Suboxone) with a total count of 499 strips of Buprenorphine (Suboxone), 45 grams of Black Tar Heroin, 175 fentanyl blue pills, 57 grams of methamphetamine, 16 grams of THC Wax, 5 normal syringes, and 1 Nokia cellphone. All illegal substances were tested, photographed and secured in evidence locker. PD was notified. K9 Unit will be run inside and outside 700 and 800 housing units." This contraband interception definitely saved lives.

In my travels as a Surge HSA, I often provided a second set of eyes to monitor daily healthcare operations. I identified medication carts and insulin syringes that were not secured properly. While strict protocols for medication and syringe control are routinely followed by healthcare staff, there are days when nurses and dental workers get busy and careless with securing pills and counting syringes and instruments. In a community clinic, this lax behavior rarely harms workers or patients. In prisons, the results can be injurious or deadly. In a case involving a U.S. Marshal Service detainee leaving a prison dental appointment:

"The detainee was trying to steal some things in the medical area. (The officer) performed a pat search finding a home-made syringe in the left sock with a black substance inside it. The test was performed and was positive for methamphetamines."

Illegal drugs have permeated both the free world and incarcerated populations. Addiction to oxycodone, methamphetamines, suboxone and fentanyl has devastated inner-city and rural communities, and feeding addiction continues within prisons. These substances, among others, are smuggled in by staff, family members during visitation, attorneys and other visitors. Some are tossed over prison fences by friends and families who quickly drive away.

Suboxone strips and other chemical substances to smoke or snort have been sent through letters, magazines and books mailed to inmates. Many prison officials screen mail before delivery and photocopy letters to be delivered to inmates. Books and magazines with discolored pages are drug tested. Many of these pages test positive for illegal drugs. Some suppliers—even when facing criminal charges for their acts—believe they are helping the inmates to cope with their addiction or manage pain. In truth, their misplaced compassion leads to frequent overdoses. Heroic, lifesaving resurrections by correctional staff administering Naloxone (Narcan) reverse many of the overdoses. In one Tennessee prison I visited, Narcan was used as often as twice daily to reverse overdoses. Suboxone is used in Medication Assisted Therapy (MAT) in many communities and some jail and prison drug treatment programs to lessen painful withdrawal from opioids. MAT helps break the addiction cycle in therapeutically-controlled settings but, when smuggled in, prolongs addiction.

Drones are used by inmates' families and friends in many states to drop cell phones, drugs and weapons into prison compounds. Drone-alert systems at some prisons alert security staff to a drone approaching the prison. The Federal Aviation Administration (FAA) and other governmental entities prohibit shooting down drones in prison air space, but drone deliveries are often intercepted once the parcel hits recreation yards or walkways.

Alcohol, known as "mash" and "hooch," is produced by inmates across the country by fermenting potatoes and fruit that are stolen from prison kitchens and meal trays. Trash bags and random plastic containers in inmate lockers are used for fermentation. The high alcohol brew spells horrible and is highly intoxicating. Drunk inmates either pass out and fall asleep or get liquid courage and become extremely violent. Fights with other inmates have resulted in fractured jaws, eye loss, punctured lungs and other injuries requiring hospital care.

Carelessness by healthcare workers in prisons have allowed legal medications and syringes (new and used) to get into inmates' hands. When pills are not used by the inmates who stole them for self-medication, they may trade them with other inmates for snack foods or to pay off gambling debt. Inmates with drug addiction problems will rarely question what they are taking, always seeking their next high. Narcotics are tightly-controlled, so most stolen pills will only deliver a placebo effect. However, for many inmates taking doctor-ordered prescriptions, the illegal drug/prescription drug interaction may cause kidney or liver damage, or other health issues. Syringes in prisoners' possession are most often used to self-inject drugs and as a tattooing instrument. Needles are also potential weapons for inmates used to ward off predators and threaten staff.

Daily "sharps" and narcotics counts by nursing staff at shift changes limit diversions of needles and drugs. Unfortunately, carelessness or staff exhaustion after working long shifts result in missing items that must be found. Many are misplaced, then found. Others are confiscated by officers from inmates during random or planned searches.

Impaired inmates are frightening to staff because the drugs and alcohol often take away all inhibition and create an illusion that they have super powers with superhero strength. They have hurt many fellow inmates in their path, but rarely themselves. Correctional officers often spray them with OC gas to temporarily debilitate them and put on handcuffs and leg restraints. After nurses assess any injuries, the inmates are decontaminated and then placed in segregated housing (or what inmates call "the hole").

One Georgia inmate was so high on meth that he climbed to the top of a basketball goal in the recreation yard and refused to climb down. During his 30-minute roost, officers debated spraying him with OC to get him down quickly, greasing the pole so he would slide down, surrounding the pole with mattresses to break his fall, or have someone climb up after him. I strongly protested spraying the OC as it burns the eyes and is debilitating. I thought he would get a head injury from the fall. While the debate continued, he shimmied down the pole and was quickly handcuffed. He spent the night in a medical cell for observation. When he awoke the next day, he had no memory of the incident.

Unconventional weapons are found in many inmates' living areas. Unsecured padlocks are often stolen and repurposed as a lock in a sock. At one of the Georgia prisons where I worked, a gang member was violently assaulted with a lock in an athletic sock by another gang member after he was found to have written a letter to the attacker's girlfriend. The victim nearly lost one eye and suffered head trauma. In a Nevada facility, MS-13 gang members turned on a fellow member, knocked him to the ground and kicked his head repeatedly until officers used

OC spray to disperse the crowd. After an ambulance transport to the local hospital and a CT scan, it was determined he had no life-threatening injury.

Perhaps the greatest challenges in our country's prisons are addressing the mental health needs of those men and women with severe mental illness and those who have lost hope and attempt suicide. I have worked with tele-psychiatrists in multiple states and witnessed delusional inmates with extreme paranoia, military veterans and abused women with PTSD, those with bipolar disorder, schizophrenia, depression, and older men with dementia. All were convicted of crimes they committed, but were they truly aware of their actions? In a world that once existed, had they received the mental healthcare they needed earlier in life, would they ever had committed a crime?

My colleagues shared a report of a suicide attempt where a wealthy inmate convicted of murdering his wife paid another inmate to inject him with drugs to end his life. He was revived and dedicated counselors talked to him frequently in and out of "suicide watch cells" to inspire reasons to live. A female inmate in the same prison was a cutter who attempted suicide many times by slashing her arms with various items. Talking to therapists and receiving anxiety medication showed promise for her well-being at least while incarcerated. Once released, with few resources, the prognosis is poor.

Six months earlier, I responded with my nurses in Georgia to a "successful" suicide where a gang member reportedly had a hit on his life but chose to exit on his own terms. He hanged himself from his top bunk using a pair of underwear as the noose and rope. As I watched an officer cut down his lifeless body, nurses and paramedics could not resuscitate him, and we saw other inmates obnoxiously celebrate his gory death. I lacked any words to express how sad this action made my team feel. We had a history with this man. Two weeks earlier, he was brutally beaten by other inmates and suffered a punctured lung among other injuries. Our doctor and nurses stabilized him and the paramedics air-flighted him to a trauma center where they saved his life.

If there is a positive lesson to learn from these sad stories, then it was taught to my colleagues and me in late-2022 when CoreCivic and many State and Federal partners agreed to start a proactive suicide prevention strategy in CoreCivic prisons nationwide. From the day an inmate arrives, they are screened medically and psychologically with questions designed to rate risk of suicidal factors. If they attempted suicide in the past or voice reasons not to live, they are quickly seen by mental health counselors. It may be naïve to think all suicides can be prevented, but they can be reduced with proper clinical focus and genuine empathy.

Chapter 9

I Saw Jesus in Prison

Introduction

One day in 2003, I walked through the Texas prison clinic where I worked and glanced into the open doorway of one of our exam rooms. I could not believe what I saw. Sitting on the exam table waiting for the doctor to return was a shirtless male patient. That was common. Yet, I stopped for a moment because I saw Jesus in the room! The Hispanic man in his 30's had the entirety of his back tattooed in black and blue ink with a beautifully drawn bust of Jesus Christ. Tattoos in prison are a rite of passage for newcomers and silent expressions of the inner man or woman for long-timers. Over my years in correctional care, I have seen hundreds of human canvases emblazoned with names of lovers and families left behind, verses in Hebrew and scripture in English, gang symbols, and swastikas, but the sight of Jesus was the most powerful statement of all.

Faith in Prisons

Working in correctional healthcare was truly a spiritual journey for me. While state agencies are careful not to mix religion into daily work life, many of the people who have careers in prisons have sincere faith walks. Their labors and mine are a calling. I saw this most clearly in the work lives of some medical staff who looked beyond the reasons why our patients were incarcerated, offering prayer and appropriate healthcare to keep hope alive. Leading the charge for spiritual health were prison chaplains who brought unwavering faith and learned over time to be ecumenical, bringing religiously-diverse inmates a little closer to God.

Nurses in corrections typically work 12-hour shifts day and night. One of the most caring nurses I worked with at Coffeewood Correctional Center was Jacqueline Assor. On each night shift, this diminutive licensed practical nurse integrated her deep Christian faith into her work life by openly praying for the lost and hurting. She prayed and encouraged inmates and co-workers as they went through tough times. Born in Ghana, Jacqueline had worked in an area nursing home, but found the prison to be where she was called. While having overseen care for her husband dying of cancer for over a year, she remained a mighty prayer warrior. After more than a decade in the correctional healthcare field, she hopefully inspired many more nurses to keep the faith.

In Texas, when I worked in prisons there from 2002 to 2004, chaplains were employed directly by the TDCJ. Many community volunteers from Christian ministries such as Kairos also provided prayer groups, bible studies and spiritual support. Twenty years earlier, in my first career as a photojournalist, I covered a bar mitzvah service for three Jewish inmates at a prison in Huntsville, TX. Grown men found beauty in Judaism and proclaimed their "new" manhood as usually celebrated by 13-year-olds in community synagogues. Under the watchful eye of a rabbi, they read from a Torah scroll and shared passages of the Old Testament.

In this book, I addressed the physical and mental health of prisoners, but I have seen many religious conversions behind bars that truly changed lives. The biggest commodity inmates have is time, and many read voraciously. Those men and women who read the Bible or Koran daily and practiced their faith's teachings found themselves better able to serve their sentences and reflect on how to be better people when released. During my time employed in Texas prisons, there was a state budget crisis and a number of paid chaplains were laid off from their assigned prisons. While each prison still received chaplaincy services, one chaplain became responsible for two or more facilities and thousands of inmates to serve. When cutting the TDOC budget, lawmakers and prison officials saw chaplains as non-essential employees.

In Virginia, recognition of the spiritual needs of inmates was a cooperative effort. Thirty chaplains were employed by GraceInside at Virginia prisons in the years I served as HSA and likely will continue for decades to come. GraceInside (https://graceinside.org/) is a non-profit organization that was created in 1920 with the support of churches from multiple denominations. About one-half of the funding for GraceInside chaplains is provided by the Virginia DOC. The rest is provided through the support of churches, denominational partners, and individuals. As contracted employees of the DOC, GraceInside chaplains provide one-on-one pastoral care to all inmates within the facilities. I worked with Chaplain Nicholas Meyer at Coffeewood Correctional Center and Chaplain Jerusha Moses at FCCW. It was fascinating to see how they ministered to Christians, Muslims, Jews, and non-traditional faiths alike. They organized religious ceremonies and celebrations for Easter, Ramadan and Passover, as well as bible studies and worship services for the 35 religions recognized by VADOC. I consider myself knowledgeable of many world religions and am open minded to different faith practices. However, when I received a memorandum from VADOC in December 2019 announcing their "recognized religions," I realized there is still much to learn.

Religions Recognized in Virginia Prisons

These are the recognized religions that can be practiced in Virginia prisons by one or more inmates. There was a previous standard of having five or more worshippers to be able to conduct organized worship, but that was modified.

- African American Church
- African Hebrew-Israelite
- Asatru/Odinism
- Buddhists
- Christian Science
- Church of Jesus Christ of Latter-Day Saints/ Mormons

- Coptic Church
- Druidry-Celtic
- Eckankar
- Greek Orthodox/Eastern Orthodox
- Hare Krishna
- Hindu
- Humanism (Religious and Secular)
- Integral Yoga / Siddha Yoga
- Islam (Sunni Muslims, Shiite Muslims, World Community of Islam)
- Jehovah's Witnesses
- Jewish
- Messianic Jews
- Moorish Science Temple of America
- Nation of Gods and Earths
- Nation of Islam
- Natsarim Israel
- Native American
- Philadelphia Church of God
- Protestants (Baptists, Church of Christ/United Church of Christ, Episcopalians/Anglican, Lutherans, Mennonites, Methodists, Pentecostal (also known as Holiness, Apostolic, Charismatic, etc.), Presbyterians, Quakers/Society of Friends, and Seventh Day Adventists)
- Rastafarians
- Roman Catholics
- Santeria
- Shetaut Neter/Neterianism
- Sikh
- Thelema (Ordo Templi Orientis)
- Temple of the Way-Out (of sin) Church

- Unitarian Universalist
- Wicca
- Yahwists (House of Yahweh).

Fewer religions are recognized in other states and most require more than one worshiper, but chaplains employed by the states and DOC contractors attempt to minister to them all and respect faith practices.

Maintaining Faith During the Pandemic and Beyond

For many of us, feeling closed in causes anxiety. Millions of people around the world became afraid, felt alone and had severe anxiety as the "new normal" from the COVID Pandemic put free men and women in a prison-like isolation. But when we shared life with friends at social distances, donning masks to protect each other, we believed a release date was coming. Incarcerated people know how we felt.

Max Lucado, in his book, *Begin Again*, put it well: "When everyone and everything around you says to panic, choose the path of peace. In this world of empty words and broken promises, do yourself a favor: take hold of the promises of God." While many of us practicing mainstream religions cannot fathom non-traditional worship, having faith in a higher power by any name clearly helped free and incarcerated people alike through the devastating COVID Pandemic that killed over 1,000,000 men, women and children in the United States.

In Georgia, at Coffee Correctional, there was a Catholic inmate close in age to me. He declined a COVID vaccine despite being high risk with Chronic Obstructive Pulmonary Disease (COPD) from many years of smoking. He contracted COVID and his oxygen level dropped precipitously. Our nurses placed him on oxygen and called 911. For 45 days, he was hospitalized in the community hospital ICU and placed on a ventilator. Over those days, at his family's request, I kept his sister apprised by phone daily of his teeter-tottering state of health once our prison clinic received a hospital update. When the patient could not be weaned from the ventilator and was actively dying, the warden allowed the inmate's sister and brother to say their goodbyes at the hospital. A community priest gave last rights, comforting the family most of all.

Epilogue

The future of prisons in America continues to evolve at a state and national level. In Virginia, Commonwealth lawmakers gave final approval on February 22, 2021 to legislation that ends capital punishment in Virginia. This was a dramatic turnaround for a state that is second only to Texas in the number of executions. Since 1973, Texas has had 576 executions and Virginia has had 114 (https://deathpenaltyinfo.org/). Democratic Governor Dr. Ralph Northam, by signing it into law, made Virginia the 23rd state to stop executions.

In Nevada, outgoing Democratic Governor Steve Sisolak in 2022 appealed to the Nevada Parole Board to commute all death sentences to life without the possibility of parole. A Carson City District Court judge blocked the action.

Nationally, in an executive order, President Joe Biden directed the Department of Justice to end private federal prison contracts, a promise he made during his 2020 Presidential campaign: "To decrease incarceration levels, we must reduce profit-based incentives to incarcerate by phasing out the Federal Government's reliance on privately operated criminal detention facilities." The executive order noted systemic racism in mass incarcerations and stated that decarcerating the prison population is a priority (Courts & the Law, Immigration, News, 1/29/21).

Having worked for State government-operated and privately-run prisons, I can attest to the fact that there are good and bad actors in public and private operations. Oversight and accountability measures by the National Commission on Correctional Health Care (NCCHC) and American Correctional Association (ACA), as well as internal quality assurance efforts, identify deficient operations and require timely correction through corrective action plans. Failure to correct mandatory standards that were violated have resulted in changes in leadership and contract reassignment. Family and attorney advocates for inmates often are the impetus for change. As with all industries, the criminal justice system needs to be regularly reviewed and updated for relevancy in decades to come. Public safety must continue to be the number one objective, but we must remember as Americans that we are better than what we have demonstrated in the past.

When we or our families are victimized, it seems appropriate to want to "lock them up and throw away the key." In totalitarian regimes, where human rights are not valued, that is a common practice. I respect the laws of our land and believe punishment should fit the crime. In the prisons where I have worked, too many cells are filled with former drug users and the mentally ill who need treatment, not incarceration. There needs to be a shift in our thinking as a society and in the courts to treat the ill, train those with no skills to be employable, and provide safety nets so further criminal activity is not an option. It's not about throwing money at societal problems, but focusing these expenditures on all aspects of underlying causes.

Michelle Alexander, author of the book, *The New Jim Crow: Mass Incarceration in the Age of Colorblindness*, presents thoughts to consider as the prison industry evolves: "Few would guess that our prison population leaped from approximately 350,000 to 2.3 million in such a short period of time due to changes in laws and policies, not changes in crime rates. Yet it has been changes in our laws—particularly the dramatic increases in the length of our prison sentences—that have been responsible for the growth of our prison system, not increases in crime."

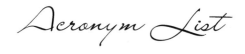

Acronym List

ACA	American Correctional Association
ADHD	Attention Deficit Hyperactivity Disorder
CDC	Centers for Disease Control and Prevention
COPD	Chronic Obstructive Pulmonary Disease
COVID	Coronavirus Disease
CT	Computerized Tomography
DOC	Department of Corrections
DVT	Deep Vein Thrombosis
EKG	Electrocardiogram
FAA	Federal Aviation Administration
FCCW	Fluvanna Correctional Center for Women
HSA	Health Services Administrator
HSU	Health Services Unit
ICE	Immigration and Customs Enforcement
IV	Intravenous Therapy
KOP	Keep On Person
LPN	Licensed Practical Nurse
MAT	Medication Assisted Therapy
MRI	Magnetic Resonance Imaging

NCCHC	National Commission on Correctional Health Care
NP	Nurse Practitioner
OC	Oleoresin Capsicum
PA	Physician Assistant
PET	Positive Emission Tomography
PPE	Personal Protective Equipment
PREA	Prison Rape Elimination Act
PTSD	Post-Traumatic Stress Disorder
RN	Registered Nurse
TDCJ	Texas Department of Criminal Justice
USMS	United States Marshals Service
UTMB	University of Texas Medical Branch
UVA	University of Virginia
VADOC	Virginia Department of Corrections

Meet the Author

Mark Elliott Miller has been a healthcare administrator, university educator and author for over three decades in Texas, North Carolina, South Carolina, Missouri, Virginia and Georgia. Mr. Miller earned a Bachelor of Science degree in Professional Writing from the University of Houston-Downtown and a Master of Public Health degree from the University of North Carolina-Chapel Hill. He also completed one year towards a Ph.D. in Applied Gerontology from the University of North Texas-Denton.

Mr. Miller's previous books include *Extraordinary Encounters in An Ordinary Life* (2002), *Advice for Life From the Mouths of Elders: One Hundred Ways to Grow Old Gracefully* (2003), *The Husband's Guide to Cancer Survival* (2004), and *The Hundred Grand Lesson, A spiritual guide for men who have lost a relationship and are contemplating on-line dating* (2007). He is an award-winning public speaker and is available to speak to groups on an array of health topics. He may be reached at professormarkmiller@gmail.com.

Photo Gallery

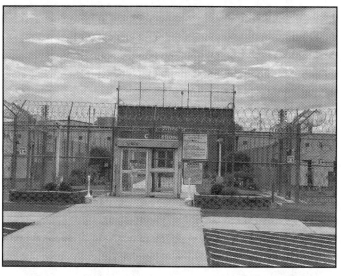

Wheeler Correctional Facility in Georgia, owned and operated by CoreCivic, is a typical design of modern U.S. prisons with tall fences and razor wire keeping the campus secure. Coffee Correctional Facility in Georgia is the same design.

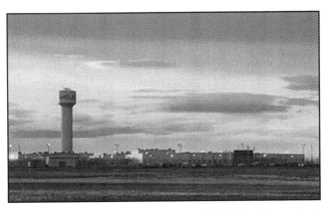

Crossroads Correctional Center in rural Shelby, Montana is a CoreCivic facility that is one of the largest employers in an area formerly dominated by the railroad industry. Prisons in small communities often increase wages in the area, offer long-term career opportunities in depressed communities, and fund improvements to infrastructure.

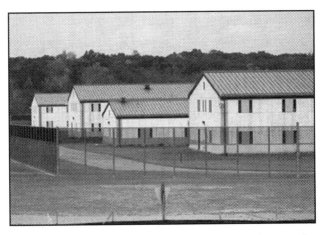

Fluvanna Correctional Center for Women in Virginia, owned and operated by the Commonwealth of Virginia, is the largest women's prison in the Commonwealth. It has been in the news and courts after the deaths of inmates.

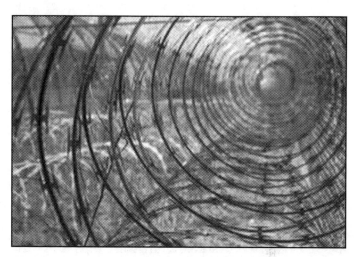

Razor wire keeps prisoners behind high fences and is an effective deterrent to "toss overs" of contraband drugs from outside friends and families. Drones carrying drugs and cell phones have effectively breached the razor wire barriers.

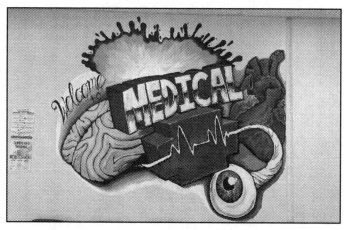

Inmates with artistic skills are permitted to illustrate prison walls. This mural in Crossroads Correctional Center is in the patient waiting room of their clinic.

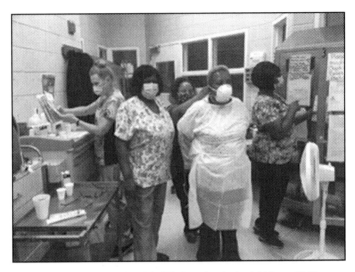

Prison nurses during the COVID Pandemic in 2020 to 2022 wore gloves, gowns, and masks with different protective levels. Proper use of PPE helped lessen the spread of COVID in prisons.

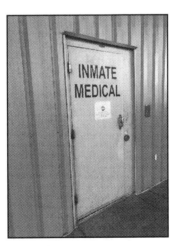

The prison clinic door opens to a small waiting area with steel benches for inmates to wait for nurse sick call, physician, nurse practitioner, or PA appointments. TVs playing movies or prison communications are in the waiting rooms of many prison clinics.

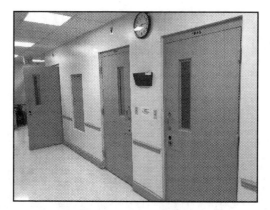

Medical Observation Units house medically fragile inmates within medical departments of prisons. Each closet-size room contains a foam mattress on metal frame, toilet and sink. Oxygen is available and individualized care is provided daily.

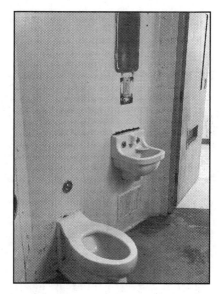

Medical Observation Unit bathroom commonly found in prison medical units around the U.S. has a handicap-accessible shower down the hall.

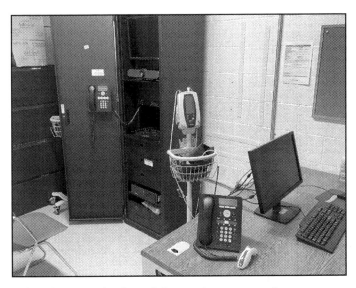

Telemedicine technology brings primary care doctors, nurse practitioners and psychiatrists into prisons remotely where there is a need for additional providers.

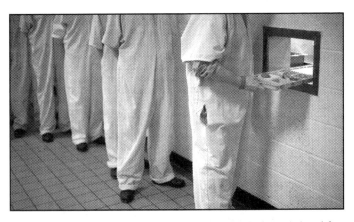

Prison meals are served hot one or two times daily with breakfast served as early as 4 a.m. Many inmates supplement these meals with Commissary purchases of Raman noodles, pork rinds, sardines, canned soda and various junk food items.

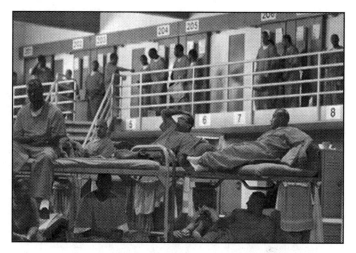

Prison housing is typically open dormitory-style for 60 inmates or more in a unit. Restrictive housing with one or two inmates per room is common for inmates with behavioral issues or in protective custody.

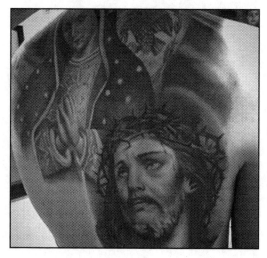

Prison tattoos express inmates' faith and love of family, as well as gang affiliations. This Texas inmate, a Hispanic Catholic, wore his faith proudly. Tattoos done in prison frequently are highly unsanitary and cause infections as serious as Hepatitis B.

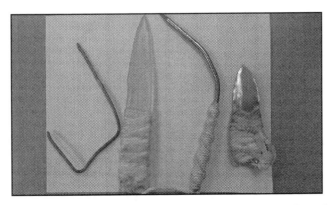

These handmade weapons were found during a cell search in the Summer of 2022 at a New Mexico prison. Virtually any piece of scrap metal or plastic, even a toothbrush, can be made into a dangerous weapon.

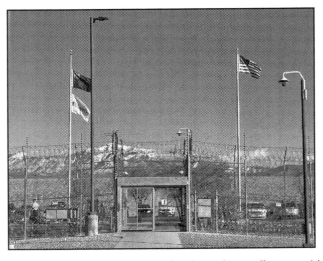

Prisons in 21ˢᵗ Century America are often located in small communities with spectacular vistas, recreational activities for workers, and opportunities to raise families in safe neighborhoods. While town residents are often resistant to prisons being in their area, correctional institutions like this one in Nevada are found to be good neighbors over time.

Notes

Notes

Printed in the United States
by Baker & Taylor Publisher Services